FUNCTIONAL FRACTURE BRACING
A Manual

Functional Fracture Bracing
A Manual

AUGUSTO SARMIENTO, MD

Former Professor and Chairman
Department of Orthopedics
University of Miami
Miami, Florida
University of Southern California
Los Angeles, California

LOREN L. LATTA, PHD

Professor and Director of Research
Department of Orthopaedics and Rehabilitation
University of Miami
Miami, Florida

◆ LIPPINCOTT WILLIAMS & WILKINS

Acquisitions Editor: Robert Hurley
Developmental Editor: Marc Bendian
Production Editor: Patrick Carr
Manufacturing Manager: Colin Warnock
Cover Designer: Karen Quigley
Compositor: Maryland Composition
Printer: Maple Press

Published by:
Lippincott Williams & Wilkins
530 Walnut Street
Philadelphia, PA 19106 USA
LWW.com

Printed in the USA

Library of Congress Cataloging-in-Publication Data

Sarmiento, Augusto, 1927-
    Functional fracture bracing : a manual / Augusto Sarmiento, Loren L. Latta.
        p. ; cm.
    Includes bibliographical references and index.
    ISBN 0-7817-3729-X
        1. Extremities (Anatomy)—Fractures—Treatment—Handbooks, manuals, etc. 2. Orthopedic braces—Handbooks, manuals, etc. I. Latta, L. L. (Loren L.), 1944- II. Title.
    [DNlm; 1. Braces—Handbooks. 2. Humeral Fractures—therapy—Handbooks. 3. Fractures—therapy—Handbooks. 4. Tibial Fractures—therapy—Handbooks. 5. Ulna Fractures—therapy—Handbooks. WE 39 S246f2002]
    RD551 .S34 2002
    6217.1′5—dc21
                                                                    2002016167

10 9 8 7 6 5 4 3 2 1

5/2/05

We dedicate this book to our wives and children, who over the years waited for us to give them more of the time we were committing to the study of fractures, and to the preparation of this report.

Contents

Preface xi

Acknowledgments xiii

INTRODUCTION 1

CHAPTER 1: FUNCTIONAL BRACING OF DIAPHYSEAL HUMERAL FRACTURES 11

Rationale 12
Indications and Contraindications 12
Management 12
Closed Fractures 12
    Open Fractures 13
Distraction 13
Shoulder Subluxation 33
Nerve Palsy 33
Manipulation 33
Brace Application and Patient Instructions 33
Discontinue Brace and Follow-Up 35
Expected Outcome 35
Complications 54
    Late Nerve Palsy 54
    Malalignment 54
    Delayed Union and Nonunion 55
    Skin Problems 55
    Refracture 55
    Limitation of Motion 55
Results 60
Basic Guidelines for Physicians 61
Basic Guidelines for Patients 62
References 63

CHAPTER 2: FUNCTIONAL BRACING OF DIAPHYSEAL ULNAR FRACTURES 65

Rationale 66
Indications and Contraindications 66
Acute Management 67
    Closed Fractures 67
    Open Fractures 67
Brace Application and Function 67

Patient Instructions 68
Brace Removal and Follow-Up 68
Expected Outcome 68
Managing Complications 68
    Synostosis 68
    Malalignment 69
    Delayed Union and Nonunion 69
    Skin Problems 69
    Refracture 69
    Limitation of Motion and Loss of Strength 69
Application of Functional Brace 75
    Prefabricated Brace 75
    Brace Application 75
    Postbracing Management and Maintenance 75
Results 75
Basic Guidelines for Physicians 77
Basic Guidelines for Patients 78
References 79

CHAPTER 3: FUNCTIONAL BRACING OF DIAPHYSEAL TIBIAL FRACTURES 81

Rationale 82
Indications and Contraindications 83
Acute Management 92
    Closed Fractures 92
    Open Fractures 93
Manipulation 93
Initial Immobilization 93
Patient Instructions 101
Follow-Up 102
Expected Outcome 102
Managing Complications 103
    Late Nerve Palsy 103
    Malalignment and Shortening 108
    Delayed Union and Nonunion 108
Initial Stabilization 109
Below-the-Knee Functional Cast 109
Application of Functional Brace 118
    Custom-Made Brace 118
    Thermoplastic Custom-Made Brace 118
    Prefabricated Brace 119
Results 135
Basic Guidelines for Physicians 138
Basic Guidelines for Patients 139
References 140

CHAPTER 4: OTHER INDICATIONS FOR FUNCTIONAL FRACTURE BRACING 143

Rationale 144
Functional Bracing of Delayed Union and Nonunion of the Tibia 145
    Results 150
Functional Bracing of Colles' Fractures 150
    Results 155
Functional Bracing of Diaphyseal Femoral Fractures 156
    Results 157
Functional Bracing of Both Bones of the Forearm 163
    Results 164
Basic Guidelines for Physicians and Patients 171
References 172

Preface

Though we have not seen the practical and effective use of new molecular technologies aimed at expediting fracture healing as of this writing, it is likely that revolutionary changes will become apparent and the means of treating fractures will assume an entirely different appearance. Now, however, surgical and nonsurgical means of fracture treatment will continue to advance in degrees comparable to those we have witnessed in the last few decades.

Enormous enthusiasm concerning the surgical management of fractures is currently sweeping the world. This enthusiasm is strongly supported by advances made in the surgical field; closed intramedullary nailing, assisted by sophisticated imaging technology, has made the surgical care of many fractures of long bones highly successful, and the procedure is rather simple.

It seems to us that the surgery, which has improved the care of many patients, has been accompanied by certain undesirable consequences. The initial higher cost of surgical care is often justifiable, because it offers a faster rehabilitation and improves the final clinical outcome. Other times, however, surgery is being performed with increasing frequency where conservative measures are likely to render the same, if not better, clinical results, and without the same time frame. These nonsurgical procedures are safer and less expensive. Identifying cases where a nonsurgical procedure would be preferable is one of the main purposes of this manual.

The emphasis on surgery in the management of fractures has also resulted in a loss of interest in the biological foundations of our profession. The orthopaedic resident in many training programs is being educated entirely on the surgical management of fractures. They no longer learn the traditional techniques of fracture reduction and plaster stabilization. They have, on the other hand, become very proficient with these surgical techniques, which eventually constitute the totality of their armamentarium.

The result of such training is that the understanding of the biological principles that govern the repair of tissues within the musculoskeletal system is not learned and never considered during treatment. This could become damaging to our profession, to the point that Orthopaedics would cease to be an important medical discipline. Today we seem to no longer be educating physicians/scientists, but cosmetic surgeons of the skeleton.

Economic considerations have entered into the field of medicine, and are being fueled by profound changes in the delivery of health care.   In the United States, we have witnessed a rapid decline in the reimbursement for services rendered by the orthopaedist. This phenomenon has made it obvious that surgical approaches are significantly more profitable for the treating physician. The preference for surgical management therefore becomes an additional incentive for the surgeon. It would be naïve to deny that financial benefits lurk at some level of our reasoning process, and those surgeons who have lost the values and altruistic tenets of medicine will abuse the system and the indications for surgery.

We hope this manual will prove to be useful to the orthopaedist, and that close adherence to the basic philosophy, principles, and technical details of functional fracture bracing will make possible the most appropriate approach to care.

Augusto Sarmiento, MD
Loren L. Lattta, PhD

Acknowledgments

We express appreciation and gratitude to the many people, who in various degrees, made possible the development of the philosophy and practice of functional fracture bracing. From the very outset of our investigations and efforts to find the appropriate place for the nonsurgical treatment of some fractures of long bones, we received the advice and support of a large number of orthopaedic colleagues, residents in raining, bio-engineers, orthotists, physical and occupational, and many others. Special thanks to the many patients who allowed us to ìexperimentî with their fractured bones, that we might identify the proper indications and contraindications for the new method of treatment.

Residents in training at the University of Miami and at the University of Southern California were the people who reviewed and recorded the clinical results we obtained with the various fractures treated with functional braces. Their support was invaluable.

Introduction

Functional fracture bracing was first described in the orthopaedic literature in the early 1960s and 1970s by one of us (8–10,11,13,14,21). This new philosophy of fracture care is predicated on the premise that rigid immobilization of fractured limbs is unphysiologic and detrimental to fracture healing and that physiologically induced motion at the fracture site enhances osteogenesis (2,7,15–17,19,20,22). These principles, however, when first advanced, ran contrary to the popular beliefs and practices of the day.

The basic premises of functional fracture bracing challenged many of the precepts that had long governed fracture management. Orthopaedists had long believed not only that fractured bones required as much rigidity of fixation as possible, but that the joints adjacent to the fracture also demanded immobilization. In an effort to eliminate the need to immobilize joints, but still believing that fracture immobilization was indispensable, the Academy of Orthopaedics introduced sophisticated methods of internal fixation. The academy added to existing plating techniques the concept of rigid fracture fixation and interfragmentary compression.

However, time has proven that rigid fixation and interfragmentary compression, rather than enhancing healing, delay it, and the callus that eventually bridges the fracture is of an inferior quality (2,7,20,22). On the contrary, functional fracture bracing is based on the premise that physiologically induced motion at the fracture site enhances osteogenesis and that through soft tissue compression, alignment of fragments can be adequately maintained (2,7,15–20,22).

We proceeded to present a few workshops to demonstrate the technique of application of the braces and felt comfortable that the published reports would be sufficient not only to appropriately explain the philosophy of the new system but to provide adequate information regarding indications, contraindications, and technical points. We were mistaken in making that assumption. Orthopaedists needed more education and detailed information on the system and its implementation. This realization came at a time when the explosion of metallurgic and imaging technology occurred and when interest in the surgical approach to the care of musculoskeletal conditions became overwhelming and was strongly marketed.

The parallel early health care reform, sweeping the United States a decade later, with a resulting reduction in the reimbursement to physicians for services rendered, further discouraged orthopaedists from a major involvement in a less financially rewarding nonsurgical approach to fracture care.

After extensive human and animal experimentation, we concluded that, contrary to popular belief, closed fractures, particularly those in segments of the body that contain two bones, experience, at the time of the injury, the maximum and final shortening (2,7,15,16,18,19). For example, a closed fracture of the tibia and fibula or a fracture of both bones of the forearm that demonstrates an initial shortening of 0.5 cm does not shorten any further after introduction of graduated weight-bearing ambulation or active use of the injured extremity. This fact contradicts the long-held perception that weight bearing on a fractured extremity brings about additional shortening (Figs. I.1 to I.5).

The current interest in surgical fixation of fractures is understandable. A great deal of progress has been made in areas such as interlocking fixation of long bone fractures, external fixation, and plating. The parallel development of sophisticated imaging technology has also greatly facilitated intramedullary fixation techniques, resulting in an enlargement of indications for surgery. In addition, the prognosis and rehabilitation of patients with a multitude of fractures have been improved and expedited. However, the surgical care of fractures is usually more expensive, a factor that reaches great importance, particularly in countries still lacking necessary financial resources. Surgical complications are usually of a greater magnitude, affecting, therefore, the cost of care. This is more likely to occur when the infrastructure of the health system is deficient.

Another reason that helps explain the preference for surgical treatment is the assumption that internal fixation is more likely to ensure a restoration of length and anatomy to the fractured bones. Though this is true in many instances, it is not always the case. For example, a candid review of the literature dealing with intramedullary nailing of tibial fractures, especially those located on the proximal or distal thirds of the diaphysis, indicates that the incidence of permanent deformity is as great as, if not greater than, that achieved with nonsurgical treatment.

Orthopaedists have been led to believe that a clinical result is best if perfect restoration of length and alignment is achieved. They also have been taught to believe that posttraumatic angular deviations from the normal are "complications" to be avoided at any cost because subsequent degenerative joint disease is inevitable. This mistaken premise has assisted in the epidemic of surgery now sweeping the world, which in turn is converting the orthopaedist into a skillful technician from the surgeon–scientist who possesses knowledge of the biological principles that should guide the practice of the discipline.

However, the scientific evidence to prove that angular deformities, regardless of their degree, lead to arthritic changes does not exist. On the contrary, there is ample documentation of the fact that even in long bones, mild angular deformities are not only cosmetically acceptable but also harmless in regard to the long-term survival of the adjacent joints. We have conducted clinical and laboratory investigations in this area, which have given us sufficient confidence in accepting mild deformities with anticipation that adverse sequelae do not occur (1,6,15,16,19,24).

The same conclusion applies to the upper extremity. Angular deformities following fractures of the humeral shaft are, unless extremely severe, cosmetically and functionally acceptable. Attempts to prevent or correct such deviation from the normal by surgical means often result in complications such as nerve palsy, nonunion, or infection.

Fractures of the forearm treated with plate fixation usually achieve good clinical results. The morbidity from plate osteosynthesis is low, and the technique necessary for its use is relatively simple. The fear of not being able to restore anatomic reduction by nonsurgical means has discouraged many surgeons from resorting to closed methods of treatment. However, attention must be given to the fact that the forearm tolerates mild angular and rotary deformities with impunity (11–13,15,23). This information is important not only to surgeons practicing in economically advanced countries but particularly to those discharging their responsibilities in an environment lacking the necessary infrastructure and financial resources.

Recent reports in the literature concerning the ill effects of incongruity and malalignment in Colles' fractures have resulted in a great interest in approaching those fractures by surgical means. Though it is true that certain Colles' fractures are best treated by surgical restoration of normal anatomy and joint congruity, only a small percentage of Colles' fractures require surgery. Mild angular deformities are cosmetically acceptable—often less noticeable than surgical scars—and have no associated functional impairment (21).

Militating in favor of surgery in intraarticular fractures is the popular assumption that any degree of incongruity leads to late degenerative joint disease. Little is known about the features present in a traumatic incongruous joint likely to produce osteoarthritis at a later date. The fact remains that mild in-

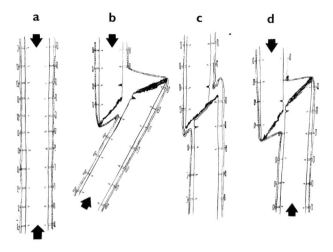

FIGURE 1.1. Schematic drawing depicts the intact bone with periosteum, muscles, and ligaments attached to its surface (**A**). An injury results in a fracture and a degree of tearing of soft tissues, proportional to the severity of the injury. The normal tissues provide a tethering that prevents additional shortening (**B**). Attempts to regain length in the presence of intrinsic instability at the fracture site create an unstable situation (**C**). When weight bearing is introduced, the unstable fracture experiences a return to the initial shortening; the intact tissues prevent further shortening (**D**).

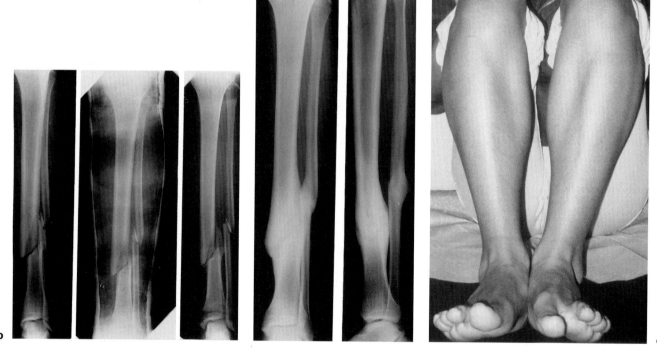

FIGURE 1.2. Composite picture of a tibial fracture illustrates the initial shortening, the same shortening in the initial cast, and in the functional brace (**A**). The fracture healed with no increase from the initial shortening (**B**). The appearance of the extremities after completion of healing is presented (**C**).

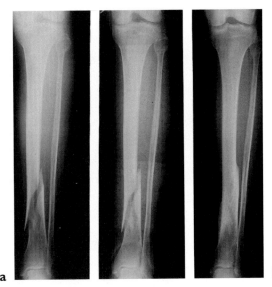

FIGURE I.3. Closed spiral fracture of the tibia and fibula is presented. Notice the minimal initial shortening (**A**). Radiograph was obtained 10 days after the injury and following the application of the functional brace. The rotary deformity was corrected at the time of application of the original above-the-knee cast. No attempt was made to regain the lost length (**B**). The fracture healed uneventfully and without additional shortening (**C**).

a   b, c

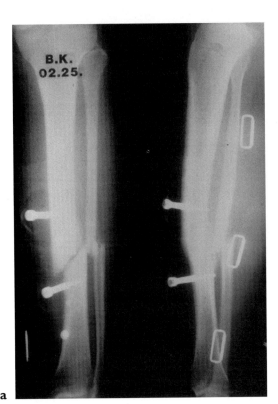

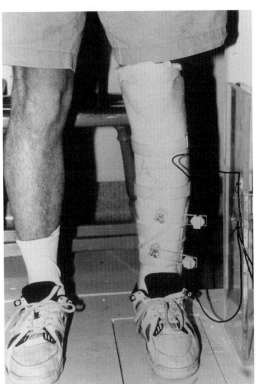

a   b

FIGURE I.4.   Radiograph of short oblique fractures of the tibia and fibula is presented. The initial shortening was accepted. Two screws were percutaneously inserted and connected to sensitive motion gauges (**A**). A functional brace was applied 1 week after the fracture occurred; the patient was encouraged to bear partial weight on the fractured extremity, and the motion taking place at the fracture site was recorded (**B**). ***Continued.***

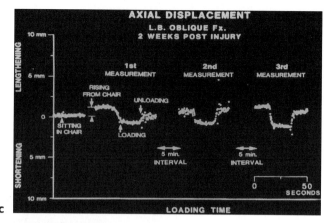

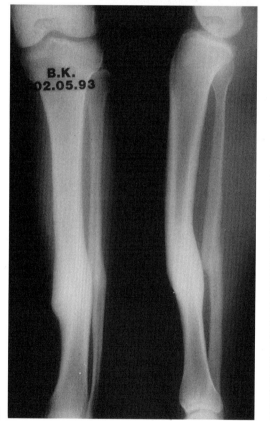

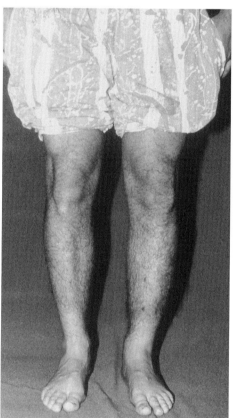

FIGURE I.4. *Continued* The recording indicates the increased shortening and takes place during the stance phase of gait but also the return to the initial shortening upon relaxation of weight (**C**). The fracture healed with minimal varus angulation and without additional shortening (**D**). Appearance of the legs upon completion of healing is shown (**E**).

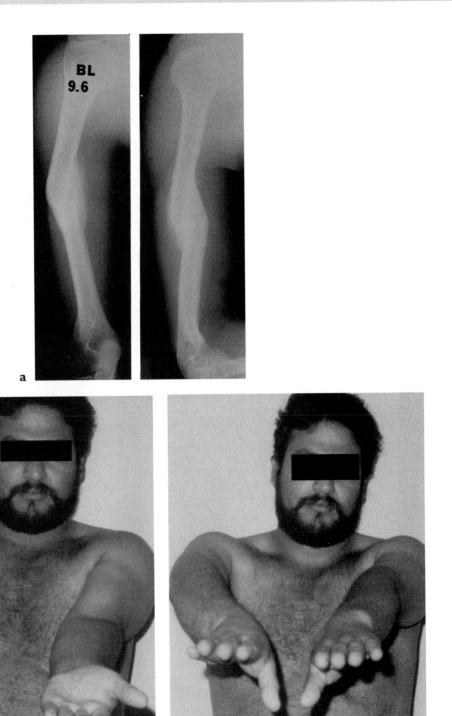

FIGURE 1.5. Pronounced varus angular deformity after a fracture of the middle third of the humerus is shown (**A**). The varus deformity appears minimal when the shoulder is in external rotation and the forearm is in supination (**B**). The deformity is more apparent when the forearm is pronated and the shoulder is internally rotated. Though radiographically the deformity is significant, there is no residual functional or cosmetic impairment (**C**). *Continued.*

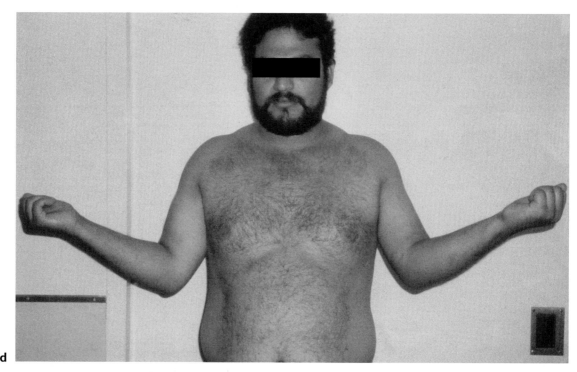

d

FIGURE I.5. *Continued* Shoulder rotation is normal despite the angular deformity (**D**).

congruity is usually tolerated well. Surgical attempts to create congruity very often result in additional damage to the joint and surrounding soft tissues, therefore compounding the existing pathology. Our own laboratory data have indicated that mild incongruous joints experience remodeling (3–5). Frequently, irreversible damage to the articular cartilage occurs at the time of the impact that produces the fracture. Surgical or nonsurgical reduction of congruity in these instances does not reverse the permanent pathology.

This manual provides the physician and other health care professionals the theoretical and practical bases of functional fracture bracing. In this manner, implementation of the new philosophy is supported, with a clear understanding of how the system works, when it is appropriate or inappropriate to use it, how and when to apply the brace, how to monitor the progress of the fracture, and when to discontinue the use of the appliance.

We initially emphasized the place of functional fracture bracing in the care of many different fractures and under a wide variety of circumstances. However, experience gained over the years prompted us to restrict its use to fewer types of fractures, not only because of failure to attain consistent satisfactory results with some of them, but because a great deal of progress was being made with other methods of treatment, particularly with closed intramedullary nailing.

The only fractures discussed in detail in this text are diaphyseal fractures of the humerus, tibia, and ulna. In a lesser degree, we discuss the rationale, results, and techniques for the use of functional bracing in the care of Colles' fractures, nonunion of the tibia, and fractures of the femoral diaphysis and both bones of the forearm. This is done recognizing that, at this time, internal fixation is often the treatment of choice, but the required modern surgical technology may not be available. Under those circumstances, the argument for the nonsurgical treatment of fractures is greater.

The cost of fracture care has become a major consideration in all parts of the world. The cheapest treatment, however, should not be the chosen one simply for that reason. Often, the more expensive treatment is the one that renders the best results and is therefore the method of choice. However, to choose the surgical treatment solely on the grounds that it is more fashionable and more financially rewarding to the surgeon is inappropriate and unethical. *Primum non nocere* (First do no harm) has been a major tenet upon which medicine was built. This precept must be preserved.

REFERENCES

1. Kristensen KD, Kiaer T, Blicher J. No arthrosis of the ankle 20 years after malaligned tibial-shaft fracture. *Acta Orthop Scand* 1989;60:208.
2. Latta L, Sarmiento A, Tarr R. The rationale of functional bracing of fractures. *Clin Orthop* 1980;146:28–36.
3. Llinas A, McKellop H, Marshall J, et al. Healing and remodeling of articular incongruities in a rabbit fracture model. *J Bone Joint Surg (Am)* 1993;75:1508–1523.
4. Lovasz G, Llinas A, Benya P, et al. Effects of valgus tibial angulation on cartilage degeneration in the rabbit knee. *J Orthop Res* 1995;13:846–853.
5. Lovasz G, Park SH, Ebramzadeh E, et al. Characteristics of degeneration in an unstable knee with a coronal surface step-off. *J Bone Joint Surg (Br)* 2001;82:428–436.
6. McKellop HA, Sigholm G, Redfern FC, et al. The effect of simulated fracture-angulation of the tibia on cartilage pressures in the knee joint. *J Bone Joint Surg (Am)* 1991;73:1382–1390.
7. Park S-H, O'Conner K, McKellop H, et al. The influence of active shearing compression motion on fracture healing. *J Bone Joint Surg (Am)* 1998;80:868–878.
8. Sarmiento A. Application of prosthetic principles to the treatment of fractures. *Spectator Lett* 1963:1–8.
9. Sarmiento A. A functional below-knee cast for tibial fractures. *J Bone Joint Surg* 1967;59:5.
10. Sarmiento A. A functional below-knee brace for tibial fractures. *J Bone Joint Surg (Am)* 1970;52:295–311.
11. Sarmiento A, Cooper JS, Sinclair WF. Forearm fractures—early functional bracing. A preliminary report. *J Bone Joint Surg (Am)* 1975;57:297–304.
12. Sarmiento A, Ebramazadeh E, Brys D, et al. Angular deformities and forearm function. *J Orthop Res* 1992;10:121–133.
13. Sarmiento A, Kinman PB, Galvin EG, et al. Functional bracing of fractures of the shaft of the humerus. *J Bone Joint Surg (Am)* 1977;59:596–601.
14. Sarmiento A, Kinman PB, Murphy RB, et al. Treatment of ulnar fractures by functional bracing. *J Bone Joint Surg (Am)* 1976;58:1104.
15. Sarmiento A, Latta LL. *Closed functional treatment of fractures*. Berlin: Springer-Verlag, 1981.
16. Sarmiento A, Latta LL. *Functional fracture bracing*. Berlin: Springer-Verlag, 1995.
17. Sarmiento A, Latta LL, Tarr RR. Principles of fracture healing—part II: the effect of function on fracture healing and stability. In: *AAOS instructional course lectures, 23*. St. Louis: Mosby, 1984.
18. Sarmiento A, Latta L, Zilioli A, et al. The role of soft tissues in the stabilization of tibial fractures. *Clin Orthop* 1974;105:116–129.
19. Sarmiento A, McKellop H, Llinas A, et al. Effect of loading and fracture motion on diaphyseal tibial fractures. *J Orthop Res* 1996;14:80–84.
20. Sarmiento A, Mullis DL, Latta LL, et al. A quantitative, comparative analysis of fracture healing under the influence of compression plating vs. closed weight-bearing treatment. *Clin Orthop* 1980;149:232.
21. Sarmiento A, Pratt G, Berry N, et al. Colles' fractures—functional bracing in supination. *J Bone Joint Surg (Am)* 1975;57:311.

22. Sarmiento A, Schaeffer J, Beckerman L, et al. Fracture healing in rat femora as affected by functional weight bearing. *J Bone Joint Surg (Am)* 1977;59:369.
23. Tarr RR, Garfinkle A, Sarmiento A. Effects of angular and rotational deformities of both bones of the forearm. *J Bone Joint Surg (Am)* 1984;66:65.
24. Tarr RR, Resnick CT, Wagner KS, et al. Changes in tibiotalar joint contact areas following experimentally induced tibial angular deformities. *Clin Orthop* 1985;199:72.
25. Wagner KS, Tarr RR, Resnick C, et al. The effect of simulated tibial deformities on the ankle joint during the gait cycle. *Foot Ankle* 1984;5:131.

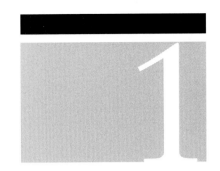

Functional Bracing of Diaphyseal Humeral Fractures

Rationale

Indications and Contraindications

Management

    Closed Fractures

    Open Fractures

Distraction

Shoulder Subluxation

Nerve Palsy

Manipulation

Brace Application and Patient Instructions

Discontinue Use of Brace and Follow-Up

Expected Outcome

Complications

    Late Nerve Palsy

    Malalignment

    Delayed Union and Nonunion

    Skin Problems

    Refracture

    Limitation of Motion

Results

Basic Guidelines for Physicians

Basic Guidelines for Patients

References

RATIONALE

Functional bracing of humeral shaft fractures is predicated on the premises that physiologically induced motion at the fracture site is conducive to osteogenesis and that immobilization of joints adjacent to the fracture and rigid fixation of fragments are detrimental to fracture healing. It is also based on the fact that anatomical restoration of alignment is not necessary in the management of diaphyseal humeral fractures. Resulting permanent minor shortening, angulation, and rotation are not complications but simply inconsequential deviations from the normal.

The humeral diaphysis tolerates well these minor posttraumatic deviations. As a matter of fact, its tolerance is greater than it is with most other long bones. Fifteen degrees of varus angulation is cosmetically difficult to detect in most instances. In heavy, muscular, or flabby people, 25 to 30 degrees is aesthetically acceptable and function is not compromised (Fig. 1.1; see also Figs. I.5, 1.32, and 1.34) (1–5,7,9,11,12).

Not all diaphyseal humeral fractures are suitable for functional bracing. Other methods of treatment, such as internal fixation in the form of plating, intramedullary nailing, or external fixation, are more appropriate under certain circumstances.

For patients with a humeral fracture to truly benefit from bracing, it is necessary for them to be able to assume the erect position, cooperate with the physician, and be capable of adjusting the brace or have someone who can provide that service on a regular basis. This is because during the first few days after the onset of disability, dependency of the extremity is necessary for restoration of adequate alignment of the fragments (see Fig. I.2) and because during the early days, the brace needs to be adjusted several times a day as swelling decreases and muscle atrophy takes place.

INDICATIONS AND CONTRAINDICATIONS

The majority of diaphyseal humeral fractures can be treated with functional bracing. Patients who, for a variety of reasons, cannot follow simple instructions, which are essential for a good outcome, should not be braced. If braced, both the patient and the surgeon must be keenly aware that permanent deformities may be greater. This includes patients with multiple injures that are confined to bed for extended periods of time and those with insensitive arms. Patients with major open wounds cannot be managed early with braces and require other means of care until soft tissue healing is sufficiently improved. At that time, the brace may be applied.

The level of the fracture is not important. The brace does not need to cover the fracture site itself because its effectiveness depends on the compression of the surrounding soft tissues (Fig. 1.2). Fractures of the surgical or anatomical neck of the humerus and those with distal intraarticular involvement require other therapeutic approaches.

MANAGEMENT

CLOSED FRACTURES

Patients with closed low-energy-produced fractures of the humeral diaphysis rarely require hospitalization. If the trauma is severe and significant swelling or pain seems to be disproportional, in-hospital observation is desirable because of the possibility of a muscle compartment syndrome in the making. This condition, if diagnosed, requires close attention and early surgery.

One of the most typical closed low-energy mechanisms of injury is a rotational force. These fractures do very well with functional bracing (Figs. 1.3 to 1.5). High- and lower-velocity projectiles and high-energy injuries may cause comminution. These fractures, however, usually do not preclude very satisfactory outcomes. Segmental fractures appear to respond to closed functional care in the same manner (Figs. 1.6 and 1.7) .

Compartment syndromes after diaphyseal humeral fractures are rare. In the absence of signs and symptoms suggestive of a possible compartment syndrome, the patient with a closed fracture of the humerus should have the injured extremity stabilized in either an above-the-elbow cast (Fig. 1.8) or a coaptation splint that leaves the forearm and hand exposed (Fig. 1.9). We prefer the circular above-the-elbow cast as it precludes the formation of uncomfortable forearm edema. In either case, a collar and cuff must also be applied for additional comfort and to minimize distal edema.

It is of utmost importance for the patient to relax the shoulder at the time of application of the sling. Ordinarily, patients are apprehensive about the possibility of experiencing pain during the application of the brace and unconsciously shrug the shoulder. If the sling is fit while the shoulder is shrugged, it is very likely that a varus deformity at the fracture site will occur upon relaxation of the musculature (Fig. 1.10).

Once the cast or coaptation splint is applied, the patient should begin exercises of the hand and pendulum exercises of the shoulder. As the first attempts to actively carry out pendulum exercises of the shoulder are likely to be associated with pain, it is best for the patient to hold the injured extremity with the nonaffected hand. In this manner, the patient, while leaning forward, swings the arm in a circular manner as well as in alternate directions of adduction and abduction and forward and backward motions (Fig. 1.11). Later, when the acute symptoms subside, the exercises can be conducted in an active manner.

OPEN FRACTURES

Open fractures associated with major soft tissue damage and significant displacement between the fragments require surgical debridement of the wound and some type of stabilization. It is in this instance when external fixation or plating is often the treatment of choice. Many prefer plating when the fracture is associated with a laceration of a major nerve or an artery injury. Intramedullary nailing may also be an appropriate treatment under those circumstances, though the complication rate from nailing is still high. However, if the soft tissue damage is relatively minor and there is no vertical distraction between the main fragments, functional bracing can be used effectively (Figs. 1.12 to 1.15).

DISTRACTION

The presence of separation between the fragments in an axial direction suggests major damage to the surrounding musculature and might lead to nonunion (Figs. 1.16 and 1.17). There are times when the axial distraction between the major fragments disappears spontaneously within a short period of time, suggesting that the soft tissue damage was not significant. In those instances, functional bracing usually renders good clinical results. Distraction is usually greater when nerve damage is present. Fractures of the humerus associated with brachial plexus injuries have a guarded prognosis. Nonunion is common. Surgical stabilization is the treatment of choice.

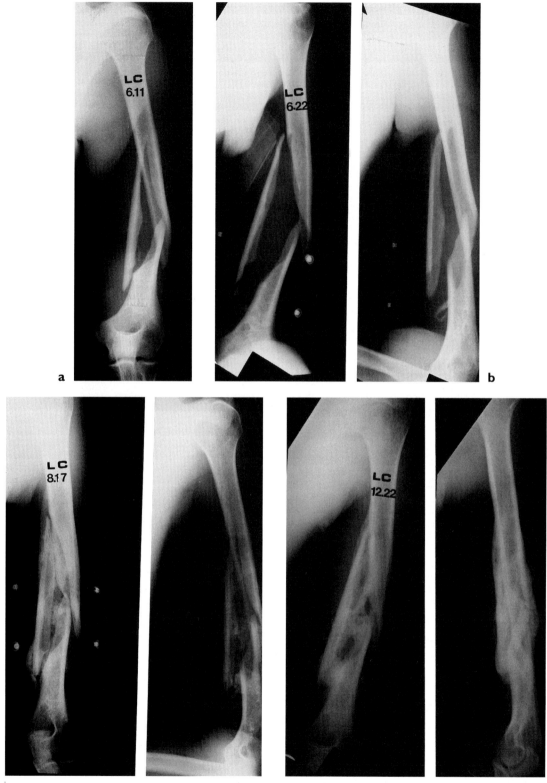

FIGURE 1.1.   Comminuted fracture with a large butterfly fragment is shown (**A**). The radiographs obtained immediately after the application of the brace demonstrate marked separation between the fragments and a varus angular deformity (**B**). Two months and 1 week after the initial insult, callus had bridged the fragments and the angular deformity had improved spontaneously (**C**). The brace was discontinued at this time. Six months after the initial injury, the fracture had further solidified (**D**). *Continued.*

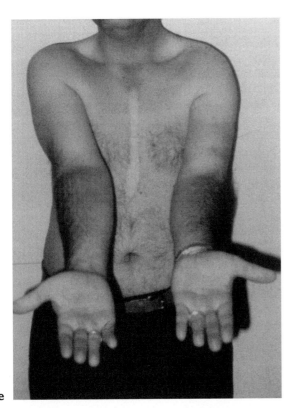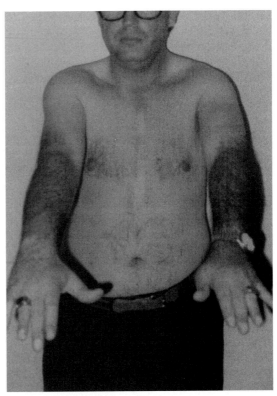

e f

FIGURE 1.1. _Continued_ Clinical photographs illustrate the inconsequential residual varus deformity (**E and F**).

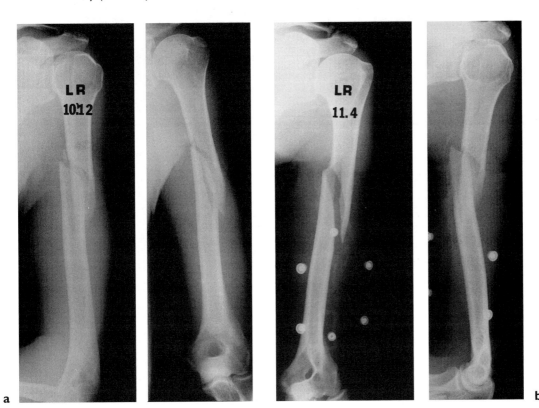

a b

FIGURE 1.2. Oblique fracture of the middle third of the humerus demonstrates minimal angular deformity and overriding of the fragments (**A**). In the brace, the fracture shows mild angulation (**B**). _Continued._

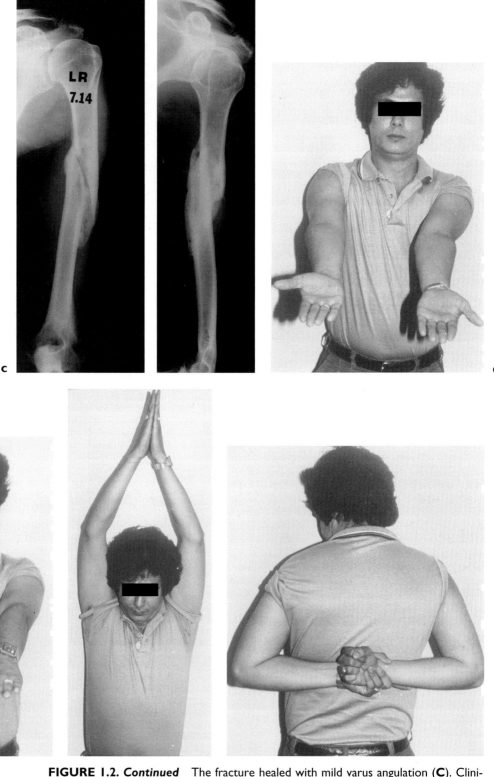

FIGURE 1.2. *Continued* The fracture healed with mild varus angulation (**C**). Clinically, the varus deformity is hidden when the shoulder is externally rotated and the forearm is supinated (**D**). The loss of the carrying angle is easily demonstrated when the shoulder is internally rotated and the forearm is pronated (**E**). The patient did not experience a loss of shoulder elevation (**F**) or rotation (**G**).

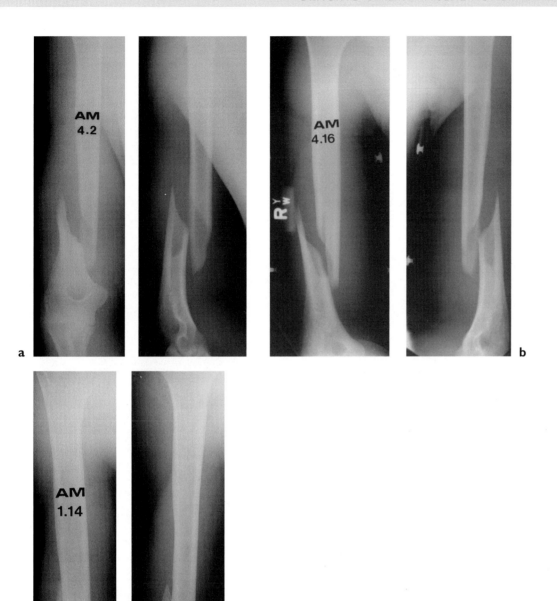

a

b

c

FIGURE 1.3. Oblique fracture of the distal third of the humerus is shown (**A**). Immediately after the application of the functional brace, the overall alignment was not improved (**B**). Continued use of the extremity resulted in an acceptable restoration of alignment of the fragments and healing of the fracture (**C**). *Continued.*

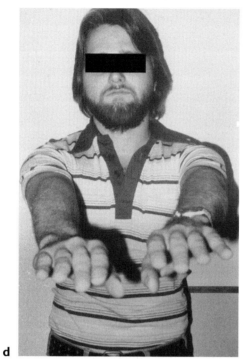

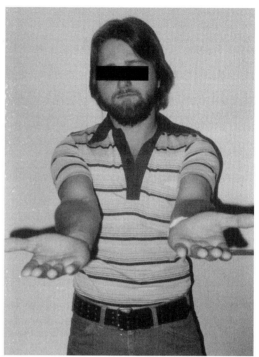

d

e

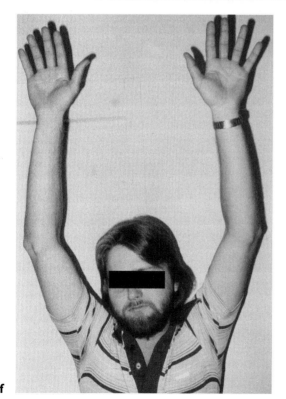

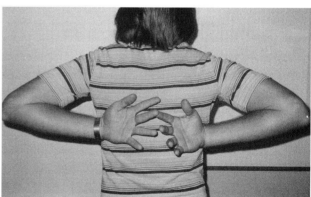

f

g

FIGURE 1.3. *Continued*   Clinically, the patient demonstrated full range of motion of all joints and good cosmetic appearance of the injured extremity (**D–G**).

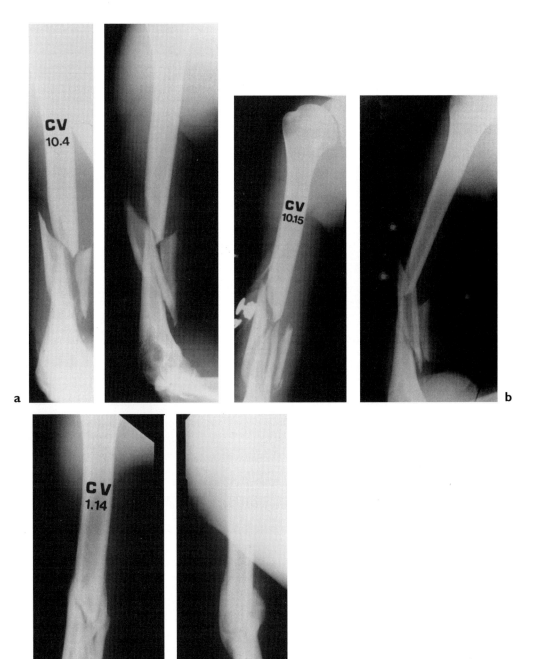

FIGURE 1.4. Comminuted fracture is located on the distal third of the humerus (**A**). Radiographic appearance of the humerus immediately after application of the brace is shown. Notice the posterior angulation at the fracture site (**B**). Three months later, the fracture has healed with good alignment of the fragments (**C**).

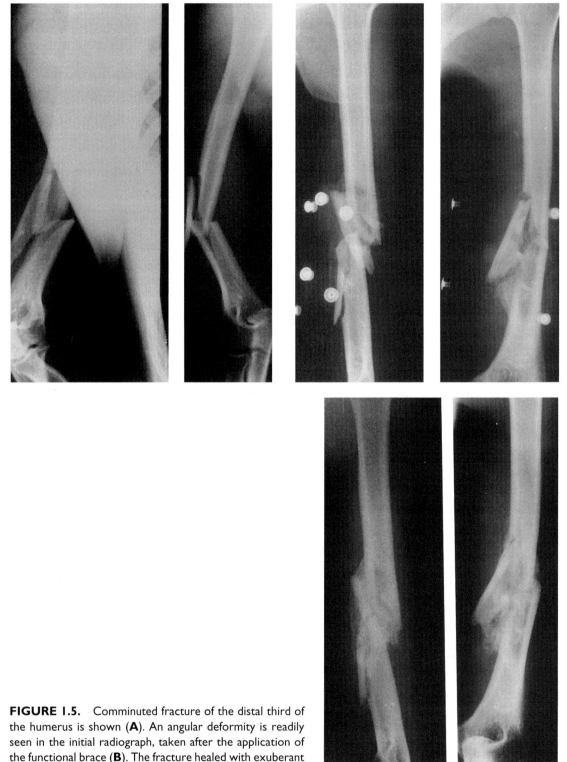

FIGURE 1.5. Comminuted fracture of the distal third of the humerus is shown (**A**). An angular deformity is readily seen in the initial radiograph, taken after the application of the functional brace (**B**). The fracture healed with exuberant callus and good alignment (**C**).

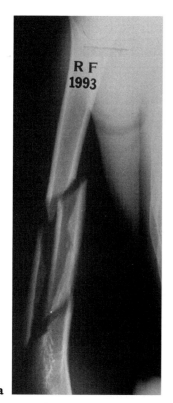
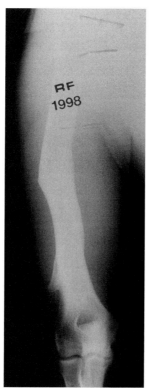
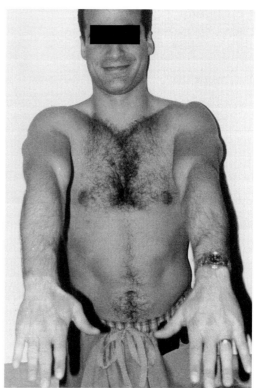

a   b, c

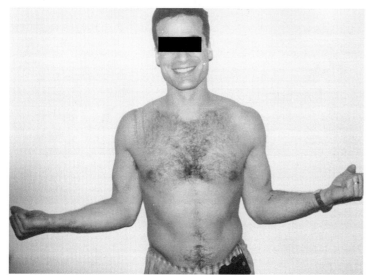

d

FIGURE 1.6.   Comminuted segmental fracture of the shaft of the humerus is shown (**A**). The fracture was treated with a functional brace and healed with a varus deformity (**B**). The patient demonstrates the cosmetic appearance of the extremity and its full range of motion (**C and D**).

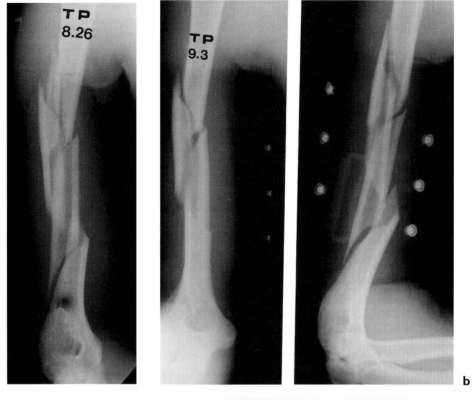

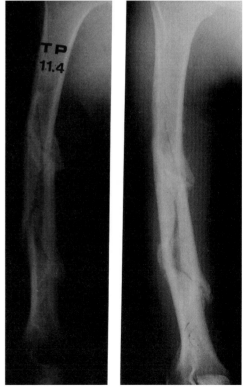

FIGURE 1.7.   Comminuted segmental fracture is shown. Notice the desirable mild overriding of the fragments (**A**). Acceptable alignment of the fragments is seen following application of the functional brace 1 week after the initial injury (**B**). Two months later, the fracture appeared to be united and in good alignment (**C**). *Continued.*

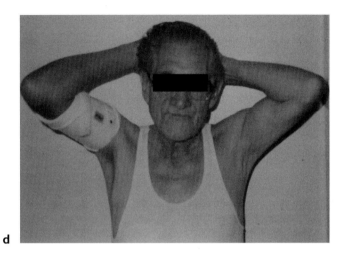

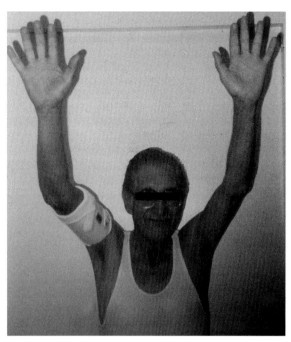

d

e

FIGURE 1.7. Continued   The patient demonstrates range of motion on the day the brace was permanently discontinued. Notice the slight limitation of shoulder elevation, which in all probability spontaneously improved (**D and E**).

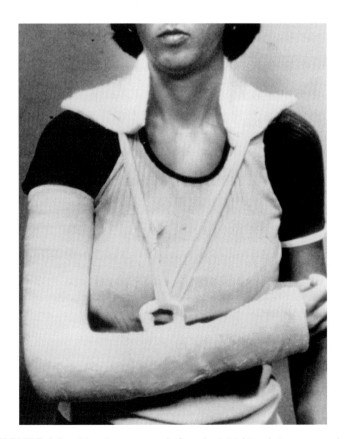

FIGURE 1.8.   Hanging cast used after the initial insult is presented.

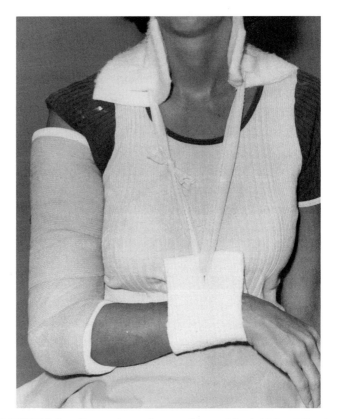

FIGURE 1.9.   Coaptation splint may be used for initial stabilization.

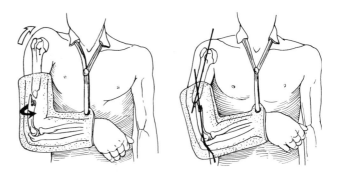

FIGURE 1.10.   Illustration demonstrates the importance of applying the initial cast and subsequent functional brace while the shoulder is relaxed. The initial shrugging of the shoulder and its subsequent relaxation produce a varus and/or anteroposterior deformity at the fracture site.

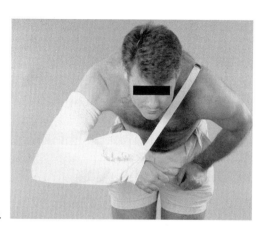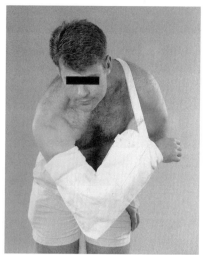

a   b

FIGURE 1.11.   The pendulum exercises to be initiated as soon as possible after the initial injury are demonstrated (**A and B**).

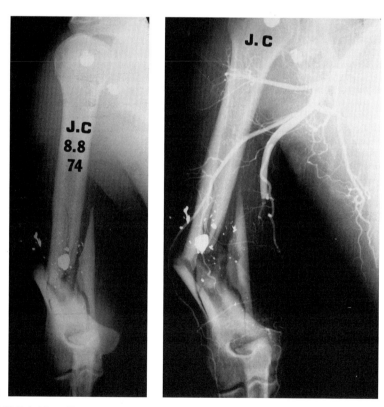

a   b

FIGURE 1.12.   Comminuted fracture produced from a gunshot injury is shown (**A**). Arteriogram demonstrates vascular injury, which was treated by surgical means (**B**). *Continued.*

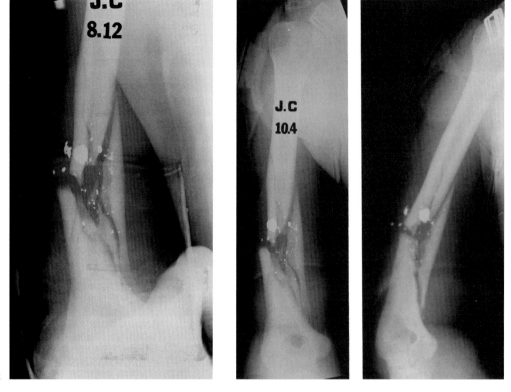

c

d

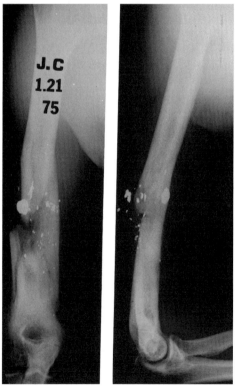

FIGURE 1.12. *Continued* (**C**). Radiograph was obtained through the functional brace (**D**). Four months and 2 weeks later, the fracture had united with very acceptable alignment of the fragments (**E**). *Continued.*

e

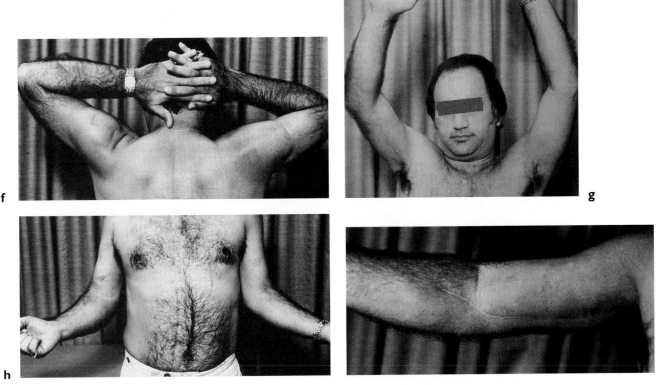

f g h i

FIGURE 1.12. Continued The patient demonstrates functional range of motion of his elbow and shoulder joints (**F–I**).

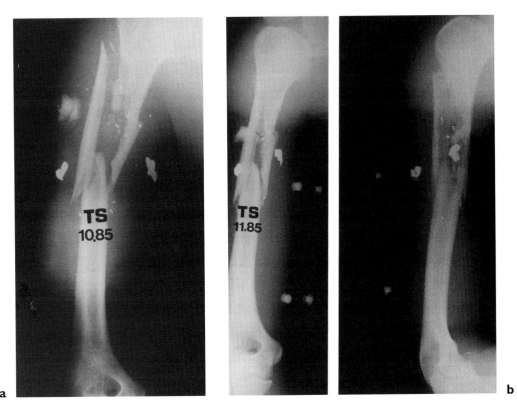

a b

FIGURE 1.13. Comminuted fracture of the upper humerus was the result of a gunshot wound (**A**). Radiograph was obtained after the application of the functional brace (**B**). Continued

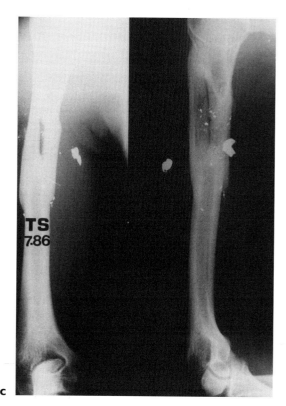

c

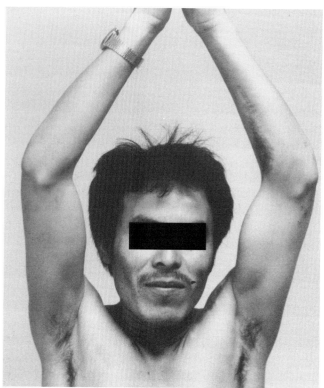

d

e

FIGURE 1.13. Continued Radiograph demonstrates solid union of the fracture and good alignment of the fragments (**C**). The patient demonstrates the degree of shoulder elevation (**D**) and elbow flexion (**E**).

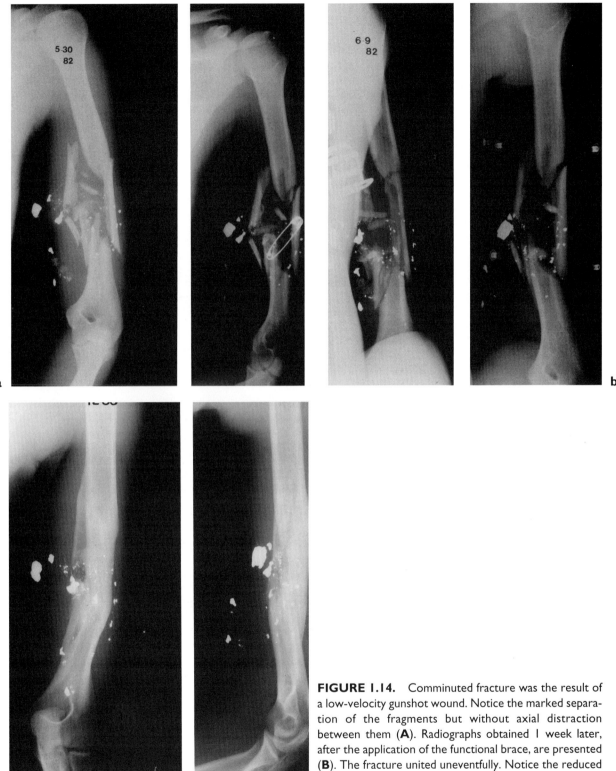

FIGURE 1.14. Comminuted fracture was the result of a low-velocity gunshot wound. Notice the marked separation of the fragments but without axial distraction between them (**A**). Radiographs obtained 1 week later, after the application of the functional brace, are presented (**B**). The fracture united uneventfully. Notice the reduced separation between the fragments (**C**).

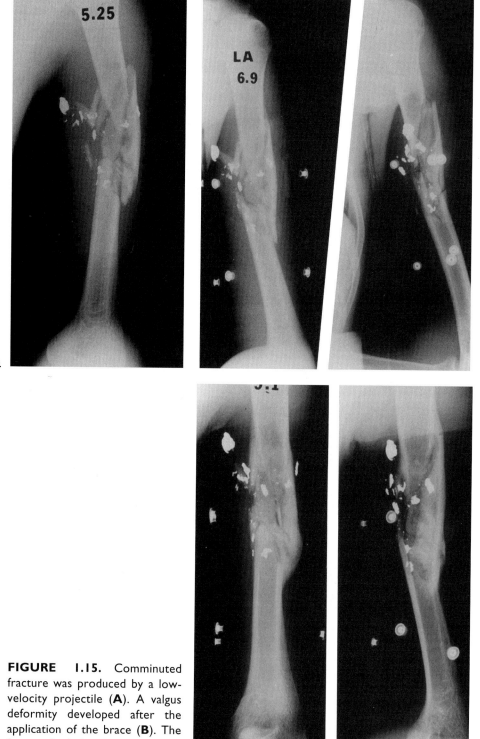

FIGURE 1.15. Comminuted fracture was produced by a low-velocity projectile (**A**). A valgus deformity developed after the application of the brace (**B**). The fracture healed without angulation (**C**).

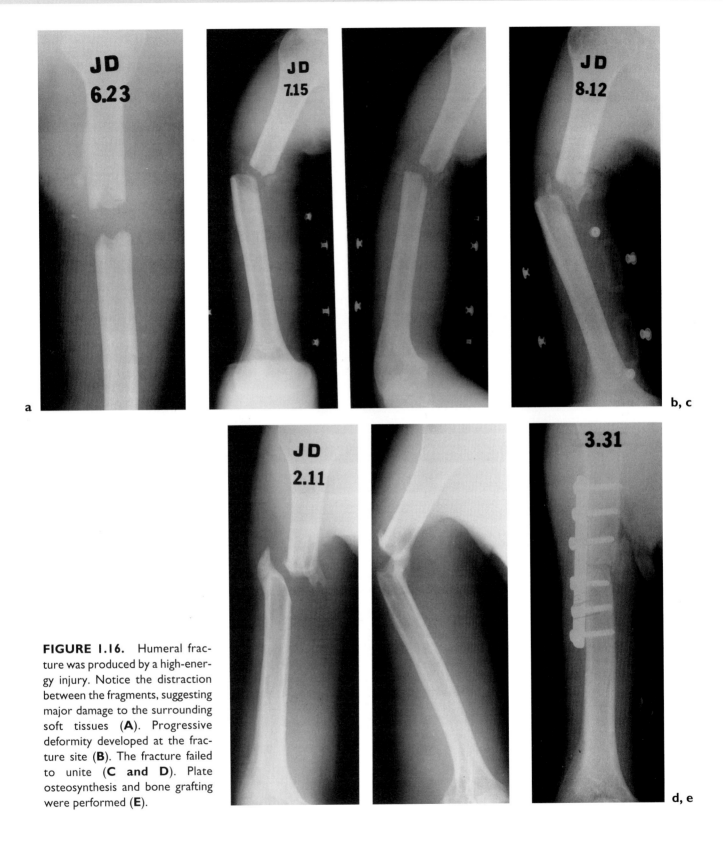

a

b, c

d, e

FIGURE 1.16. Humeral fracture was produced by a high-energy injury. Notice the distraction between the fragments, suggesting major damage to the surrounding soft tissues (**A**). Progressive deformity developed at the fracture site (**B**). The fracture failed to unite (**C and D**). Plate osteosynthesis and bone grafting were performed (**E**).

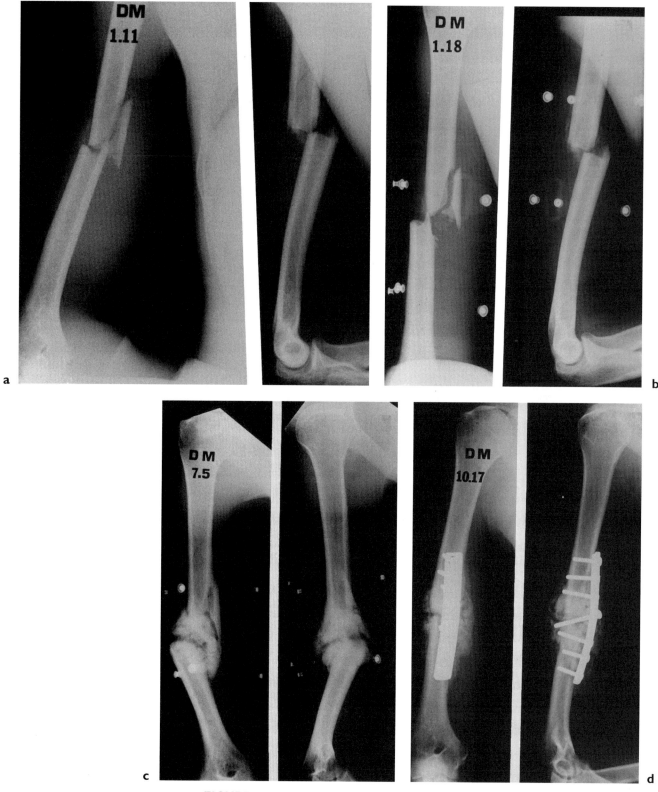

FIGURE 1.17.   Comminuted fracture was the result of a high-energy injury (**A**). The distraction between the fragments can be seen through the brace (**B**). The fracture failed to unite (**C**) and was treated with plate osteosynthesis (**D**).

SHOULDER SUBLUXATION

Subluxation of the glenohumeral joint is common after the initial stabilization of diaphyseal humeral fractures, particularly in those located in the proximal third of the bone. It is best managed by active flexion and extension of the elbow. Since both flexors and extensors muscles have attachments on the scapula and distal humerus, their contraction forces the humeral head into the glenoid (Fig.1. 18). Attempts to obtain reduction through abduction exercises, in anticipation of having the deltoid muscle be the correcting force, may result in the production of a varus deformity at the fracture site.

NERVE PALSY

Radial palsy is frequently associated with diaphyseal humeral fractures. In our series, the incidence of radial palsy was 11%. Most closed fractures with associated radial palsy may be treated with functional bracing in anticipation of spontaneous recovery (Fig. 1.19). This is true especially if the nerve palsy develops immediately after the injury.

A dorsal cock-up wrist splint is not usually necessary if no contraindications exist for early extension of the elbow. Once the elbow is extended, the partially paralyzed wrist spontaneously extends, preventing, in that manner, the development of a flexion contracture of the joint. Passive extension and abduction of the thumb should be carried out with the opposite hand to prevent an adduction contracture of the digit.

If the palsy appears at a later day, the prognosis is more guarded because it suggests encroachment of the nerve by the forming callus. This is an unusual complication with closed functional bracing but a common one after plating or intramedullary nailing. Whenever late palsy appears, magnetic resonance imaging (MRI) and electrical studies should be conducted to rule out the possibility of serious pathology. If identified, surgical exploration is necessary.

After the repair of the nerve, the fractured humerus should be stabilized with either an external fixator, a plate, or an intramedullary nail.

MANIPULATION

Manipulation of diaphyseal fractures of the humerus is strongly criticized because of the danger of producing nerve damage. Most angular deformities correct spontaneously as the brace compresses the soft tissues and the weight of the arm assists in improving alignment (Figs. 1.20 and 1.21). Most angular deformities are physiologically and cosmetically tolerated. If the conservative approach fails to provide the desired alignment of the fragments, a surgical intervention is required.

BRACE APPLICATION AND PATIENT INSTRUCTIONS

The brace should not be used as the initial means of stabilization because it is likely to create uncomfortable distal extremity swelling and pain. A cast or coaptation splint performs better.

The brace must be adjustable; otherwise, it does not make possible the maintenance of firm compression of the soft tissues surrounding the fractured humerus. It is the snug fit of the brace that provides comfort to the patient and permits the continued use of the injured extremity in a gradually progressive manner.

The brace can be prefabricated or custom-made. A circular brace that is not adjustable cannot be kept in place without slipping distally as the initial swelling decreases and muscle atrophy takes place. The material used can be either plastic or plaster of Paris. A "soft plaster," currently used in Europe, is lighter and easier to keep in place than the heavier regular plaster. Regardless of the material used, Velcro straps or similar mechanisms ensure the adjustability of the brace.

The brace should extend from approximately 1 in below the axilla to approximately 1 in above the humeral epicondyles. It does not have to extend above and below the fracture site. The important thing is the compression of the soft tissues around the fracture site. The sleeve should not extend over the acromion or the epicondyles of the humerus or be suspended with a harness over the shoulder.

The proximal extension over the acromion does not add to the effectiveness of the sleeve. In addition, it can do harm by wrongly suggesting that in this manner the sleeve does not displace distally and provides greater stabilization to the fractured humerus. The extension of the brace over the epicondyles is also an exercise in futility as in order for the condyles to prevent its distal slippage, a significant amount of pressure over the skin will be necessary—a degree of pressure that can lead to pain and pressure sores.

It is possible, in most instances, to exchange the cast for a functional brace between the end of the first and second weeks after injury. This period of time is usually required for the subsidence of acute symptoms and the patient's ability to carry out the above-described exercises.

Whenever possible, the initial cast should be removed while the patient sits on a high table. The brace is applied in the same position. After the arm is cleansed, a layer of stockinet is carefully rolled over the extremity, extending from just below the elbow to the level of the acromial process. The appropriate size of the brace is selected by measuring the length of the upper arm from approximately 1 in below the axilla to just above the lateral condyle of the humerus (Fig. 1.22A–D).

The brace should not press superiorly against the axilla because it will produce discomfort and sufficient pressure to lacerate the skin and force the patient to hold the arm in an abducted position. A varus angular deformity will then occur. The collar and cuff are applied, with the elbow held at 90 degrees.

The brace is applied to the arm and tightened to compress the soft tissues. The stockinet can be reflected back over the proximal and distal edges of the brace (Fig. 1.22F–G).

Exercises similar to those carried out during the cast immobilization period should continue. At first, they should be passively assisted with the opposite hand (Fig. 1.23A–C). As soon as the patient realizes that the passive motion of the shoulder is not associated with pain, he or she should begin to combine the passive motion with active contraction of the biceps and triceps.

The contraction of the flexors and extensors of the elbow assists in the correction of rotary deformities. This is possible because the two muscle groups have attachments to the proximal and distal fragments of the fracture. The malrotation of the bones at the time of the injury is accompanied by a parallel coiling of the muscles. Once they contract, they correct the rotary bony deformity (Fig. 1.24).

Patients should be instructed to continue pendulum exercises and to begin passive elbow extension with the sling removed (Fig. 1.23C–G). The arm must hang loosely at the side of the body in order for gravity forces to assist in the correction of angular deformities.

As symptoms subside and the patient is comfortable with elbow extension, the sling should be worn only at night.

The exercises of the extremity should not be limited to the shoulder and elbow and should include the hand and wrist. Swelling is decreased in this manner.

Compression of the soft tissues by the brace is essential for the maintenance of fracture alignment and stabilization of the fragments. It is important, therefore, to use adjustable braces. As swelling subsides and muscle atrophy experiences recovery, the need for frequent adjustment of the brace decreases. Patients should be instructed to remove the brace for hygiene and after bathing (Fig. 1.25). The stockinet is replaced with clean, dry stockinet, and the brace is reapplied.

Active abduction and elevation of the arm should be avoided until there is radiographic evidence of early healing. Therefore, only passive exercises and active ones that do not call for strong contraction of the abductors and elevators of the shoulder should be conducted. Once intrinsic stability at the fracture occurs, active elevation and abduction may be conducted (Fig. 1.26). If physical and/or occupational therapy exercises are prescribed, they should be limited to the exercises described above. In most instances, supervised rehabilitation is not needed.

It is not necessary for the patient to sleep in the sitting position. All that is needed is the suspension of the arm in the sling. It is most desirable to regain extension of the elbow in preference to flexion as it is anticipated that with the necessary activities of daily living, spontaneous gain of flexion will take place. Regaining extension early is important because once full extension of the elbow is reached, the patient can discontinue the use of the sling and walk with the swing of the arm in a normal way. The weights of the distal arm can now further assist in improving the ubiquitous varus angulation seen in humeral diaphyseal fractures (Figs. 1.27 to 1.29).

In addition, the extension of the elbow eliminates the fulcrum effect created by the chest when the arm rests over protruding muscular tissues or large breasts. It is well known that large-breasted women have a greater tendency to develop varus deformities as a result of the alleged fulcrum effect (see Figs. I.5 and 1.27).

DISCONTINUE USE OF BRACE AND FOLLOW-UP

The brace is permanently discontinued when clinical and radiologic evidence of union is documented. The absence of pain and the presence of osseous bridging of the fragments indicate union. Patients should continue to exercise their joints and to rebuild the musculature of the arm. Strenuous exercises such as sporting activities that require maximum force should be introduced gradually. Failure to follow such a protocol may result in refracture (Figs. 1.30 and 1.31).

EXPECTED OUTCOME

Eventual return of normal motion of the shoulder and elbow joints should be expected in the overwhelming majority of instances. If a major deformity at the fracture site becomes permanent as a result of inappropriate use of the brace and extremity, a permanent limitation of motion of the elbow may result. Deformities of this degree are preventable and more likely to develop in transverse, nondisplaced fractures (Figs. 1.32 and 1.33).

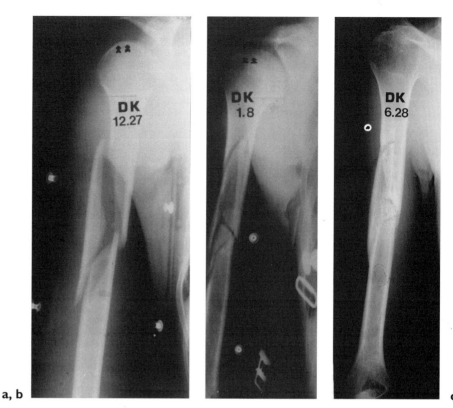

a, b   c

FIGURE 1.18. Radiograph of a comminuted fracture was taken a few days after the initial injury. Notice subluxation of the glenohumeral joint (**A**). The subluxation improved rapidly after the initiation of active contractions of the elbow flexor and extensor muscles (**B**). The fracture healed uneventfully (**C**).

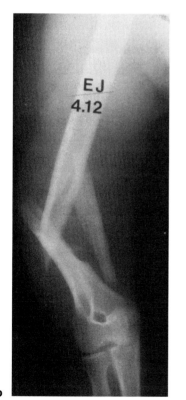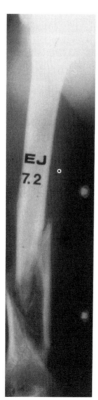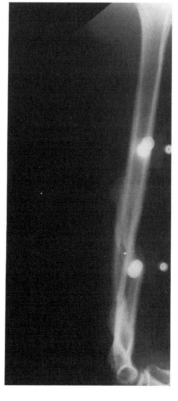

FIGURE 1.19. Comminuted extra-articular fracture of the distal humerus demonstrates the frequently seen medial butterfly fragment (**A**). After application of the brace and the introduction of pendulum exercises, the alignments of the fragments improved spontaneously (**B**). *Continued.*

a, b

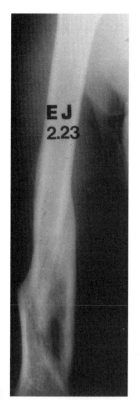

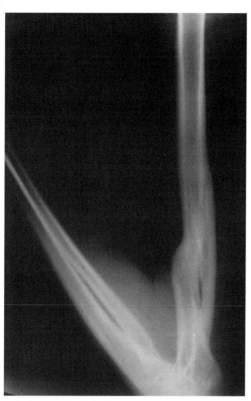

c

d

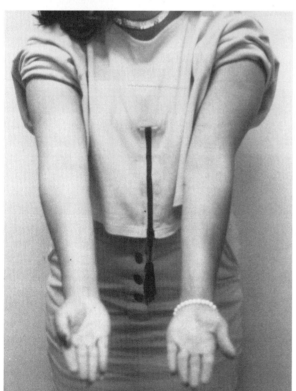

e

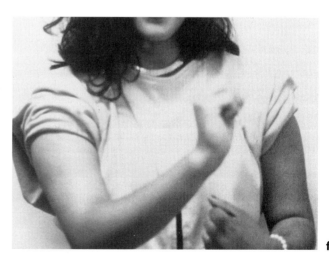

f

FIGURE 1.19. *Continued* The fracture united with acceptable alignment (**C and D**). The mild residual loss of the "carrying angle" was cosmetically and functionally acceptable (**E**). The radial palsy improved spontaneously (**F**).

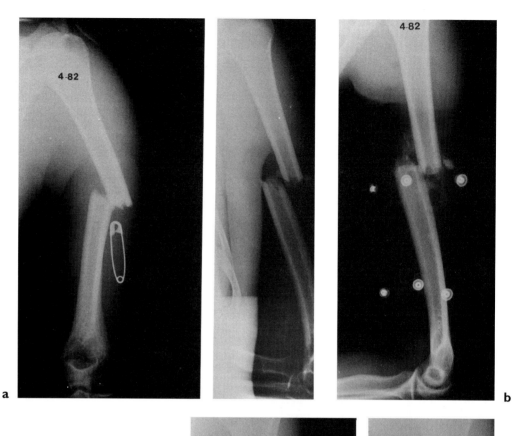

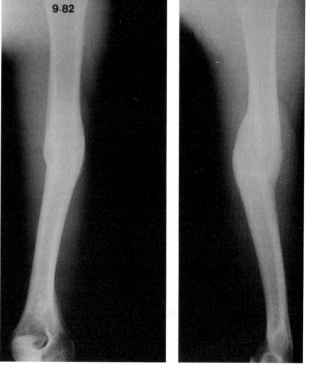

FIGURE 1.20. Transverse fracture in the middle third of the humerus with overriding of the fragments is shown (**A**). The alignment of the fragments improved after application of the functional brace (**B**). The fracture healed with a mild angular deformity (**C**). *Continued.*

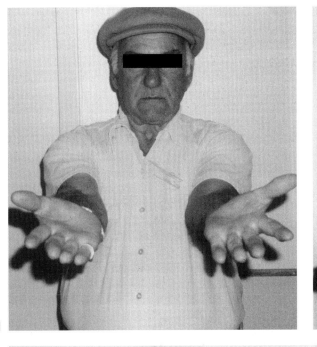
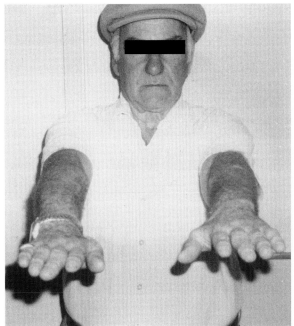

d

e

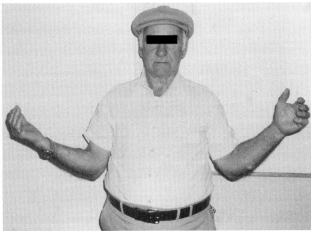
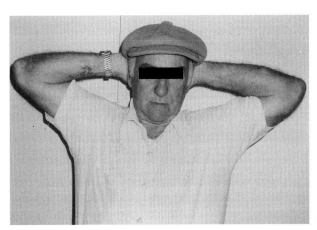

f

g

FIGURE 1.20. *Continued* The patient demonstrates the cosmetic appearance of the extremity and the function of his joints (**D–G**).

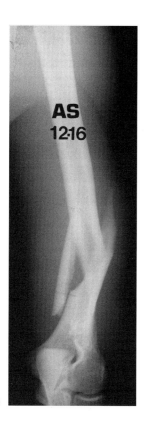
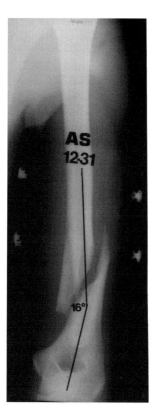
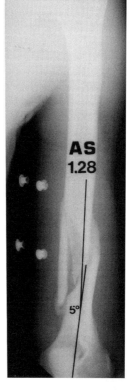

a, b

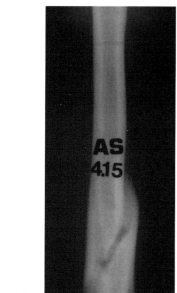
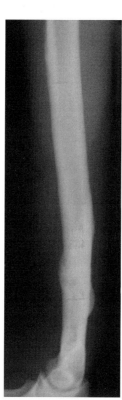

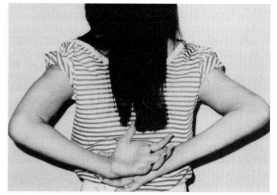

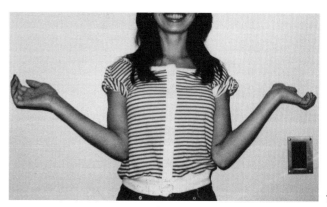

c. d

e

f

FIGURE 1.21. Closed comminuted fracture of the distal third of the humerus demonstrates a frequently seen medial fragment and varus angulation (**A**). After the application of the brace and dependency of the extremity, the angulation improved (**B**). One month later, further improvement in alignment and early callus can be seen (**C**). Upon completion of healing, the overall alignment of the fragments is good (**D**). Clinical appearance and range of motion of the shoulder and elbow after completion of healing are shown (**E, F**).

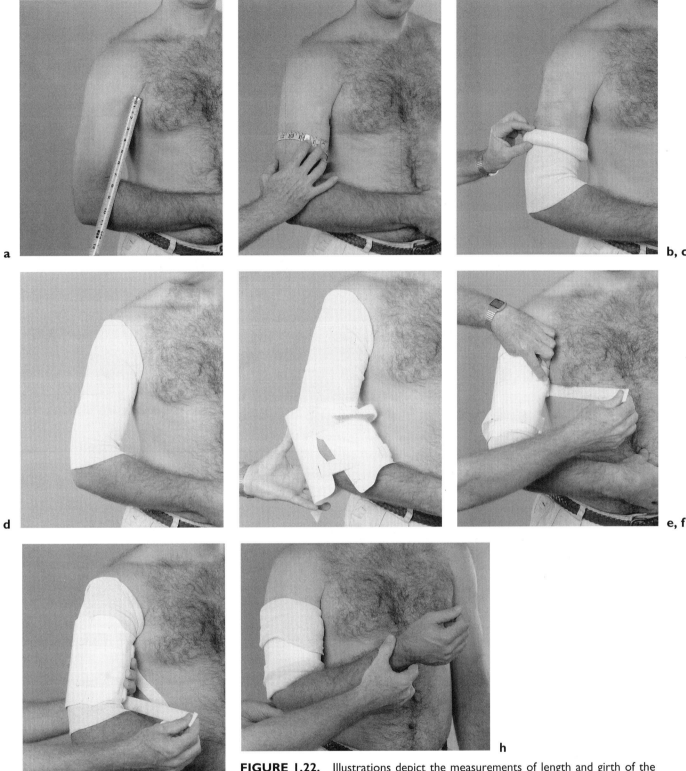

FIGURE 1.22. Illustrations depict the measurements of length and girth of the upper arm to determine the appropriate size of the functional brace (**A and B**), the rolling of the stockinet (**C and D**), the application of the brace and tightening of the Velcro straps (**E–G**), and initial passive range of motion of the elbow (**H**).

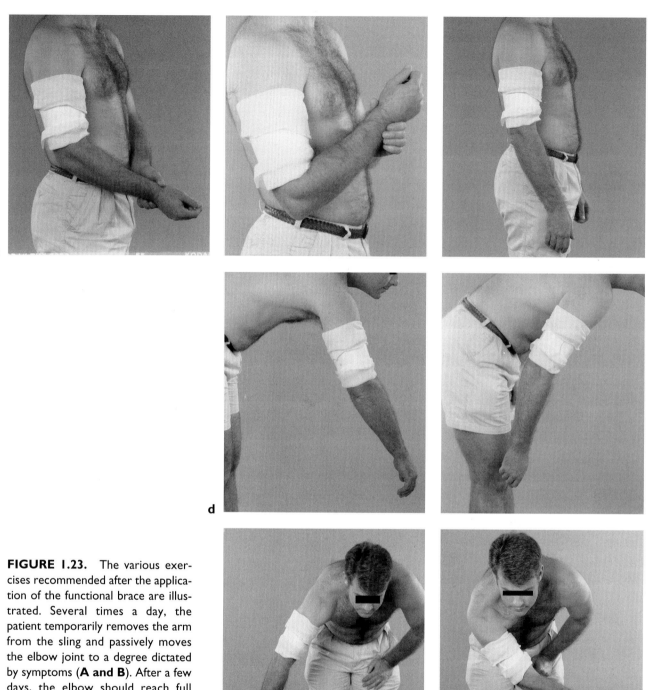

a, b

c

d

e

FIGURE I.23. The various exercises recommended after the application of the functional brace are illustrated. Several times a day, the patient temporarily removes the arm from the sling and passively moves the elbow joint to a degree dictated by symptoms (**A and B**). After a few days, the elbow should reach full extension (**C**). Then, with the elbow extended, the pendulum exercises are continued (**D and E**). Similar abduction and adduction exercises should also be conducted (**F and G**).

f

g

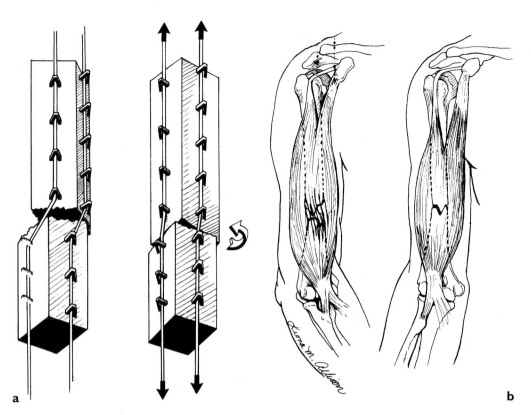

a   b

FIGURE 1.24. The possible mechanism that corrects rotary deformities is illustrated. The rotation of the bony fragments that occurs at the time of the injury is associated with a similar coiling of the surrounding musculature. When the flexor and extensor of the elbow contract, uncoiling occurs and the initial rotary deformity is partially corrected (**A and B**).

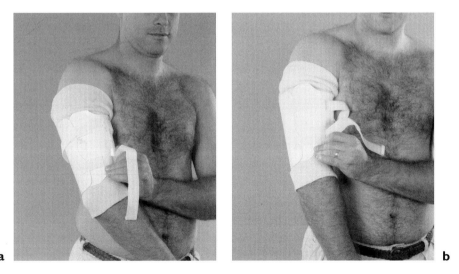

a   b

FIGURE 1.25. Patients should be instructed to remove the brace for hygiene and after bathing (**A–D**). *Continued.*

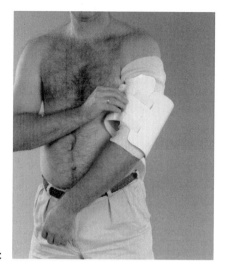

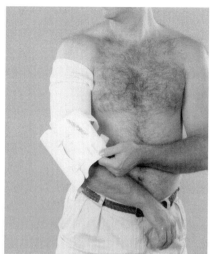

c

d

FIGURE 1.25. *Continued*

FIGURE 1.26.   Active elevation exercises to the shoulder *should not* be performed before the presence of intrinsic stability at the fracture site (**A**). As soon as intrinsic stability of the fragments is suspected, abduction and elevation of the shoulder may be carried out (**B and C**).

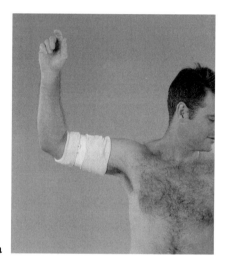

a

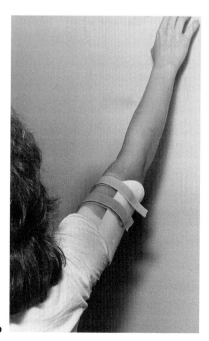

b

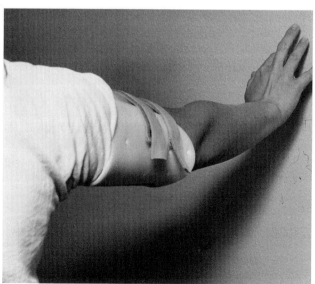

c

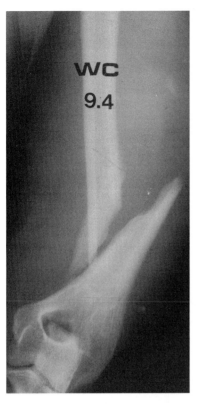
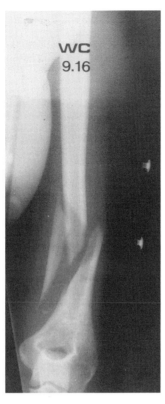
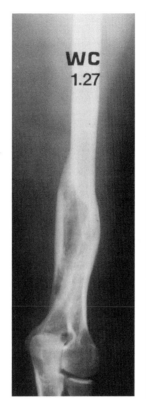
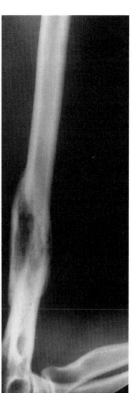

a, b   c

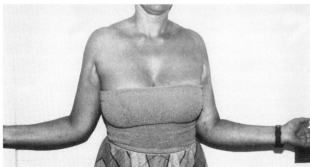

d

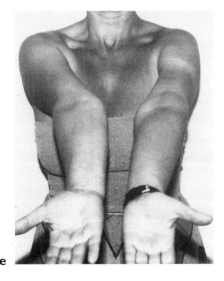

FIGURE 1.27.   Comminuted fracture of the distal third of the humerus with severe varus deformity is shown (**A**). Radiographs obtained 3 weeks after the injury demonstrate spontaneous correction of the deformity, following the application of the brace and dependency of the extremity (**B**). Radiographs illustrate the solidly united fracture with mild varus deformity (**C**). Clinical photographs depict the overall alignment of the upper extremities. Notice the inconsequential loss of the "carrying angle" (**D and E**).

e

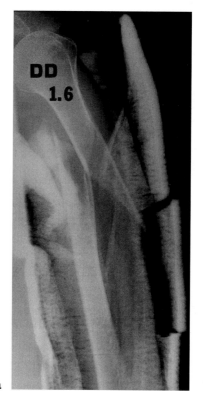

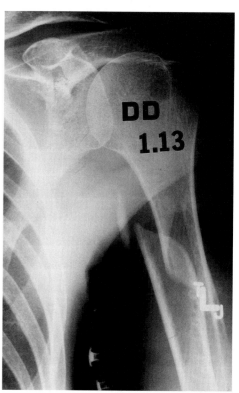

a

b

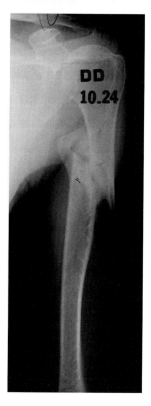

FIGURE 1.28.   Fracture of the proximal humerus is shown. Notice the severe varus angular deformity (**A**). The alignment of the fragments improved with the use of the functional brace (**B**). The fracture healed with acceptable angular deformity (**C**). *Continued*

c

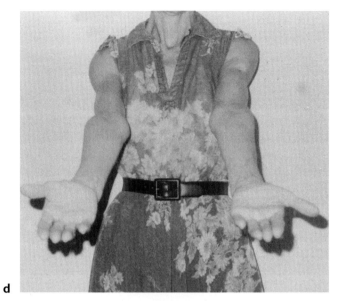

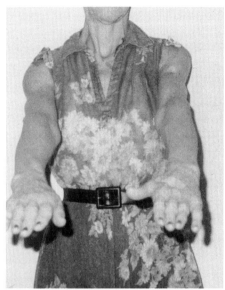

d

e

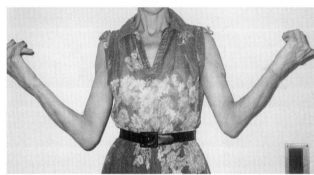

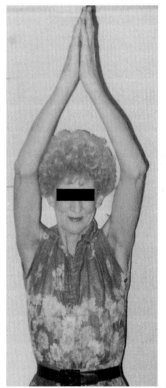

f

g

FIGURE 1.28. *Continued* The patient demonstrates the cosmetic appearance of the extremity and the range of motion of the shoulder (**D–G**).

FIGURE 1.29. Oblique fracture of the proximal third of the humerus is associated with a valgus angular deformity (**A**). Gravity forces that come into being after the application of the brace and dependency of the extremity corrected the angular deformity (**B**). The fracture healed with very acceptable alignment (**C and D**).

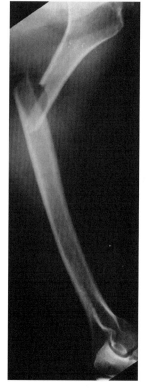
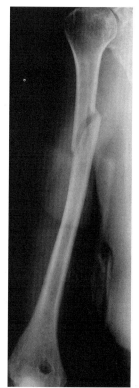

a

b

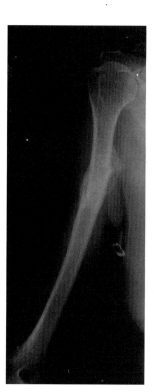
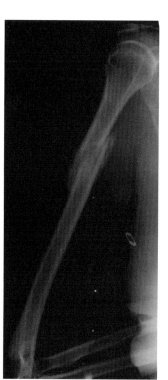
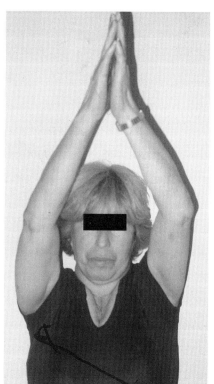

c

d

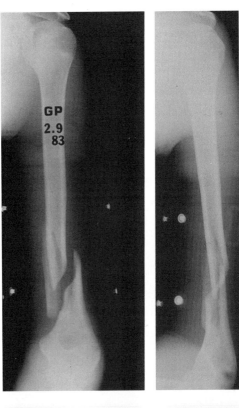

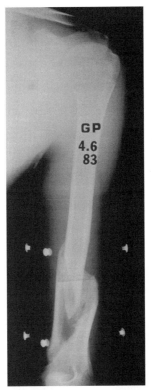

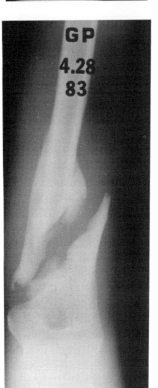

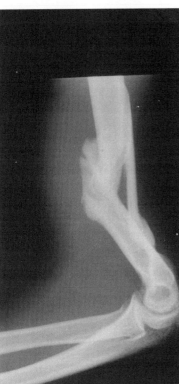

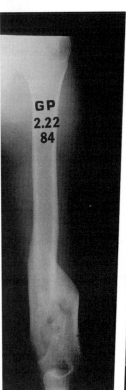

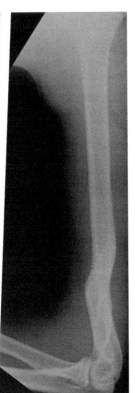

a

b

c

d

FIGURE 1.30. Comminuted fracture of the distal third of the humerus was treated with a functional brace (**A**). The fracture was progressing toward healing (**B**). The patient attempted to play baseball and refractured his humerus (**C**). The brace was reapplied, and the fracture healed uneventfully (**D**).

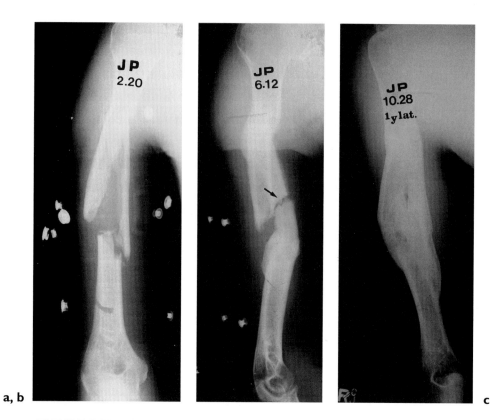

a, b   c

FIGURE 1.31. Comminuted fracture of the middle third of the humerus is shown (**A**). Healing progressed, but a new injury produced a refracture (**B**). The brace was reapplied, and the fracture healed uneventfully (**C**).

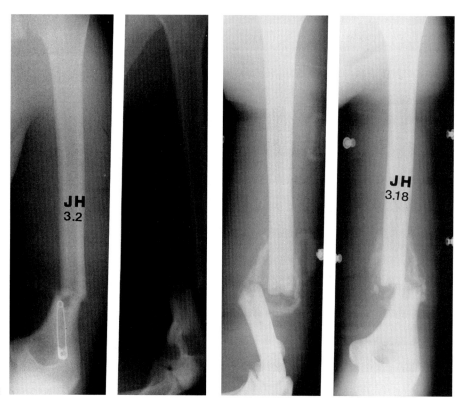

a, b

FIGURE 1.32. Transverse fracture of the distal third of the humerus is shown (**A**). Radiographs obtained 16 days after the initial injury demonstrate abundant callus and a marked anterior and varus angulation (**B**). *Continued*

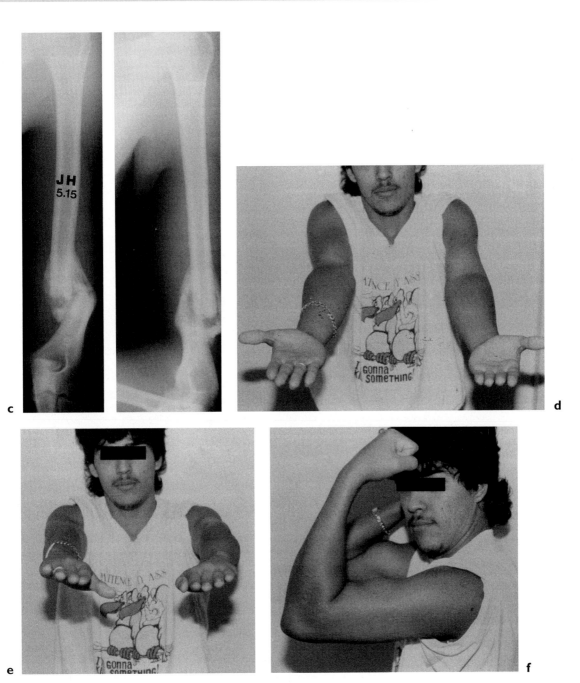

FIGURE 1.32. Continued The angular deformity was probably due to the fact that the patient frequently leaned on the elbow. Ten weeks after the initial insult, the fracture had healed solidly with an "unacceptable" deformity (**C**). Photographs illustrate the loss of the normal "carrying angle" and the limitation of flexion of the elbow (**D–F**). Transverse fractures are the ones most likely to develop angular deformities.

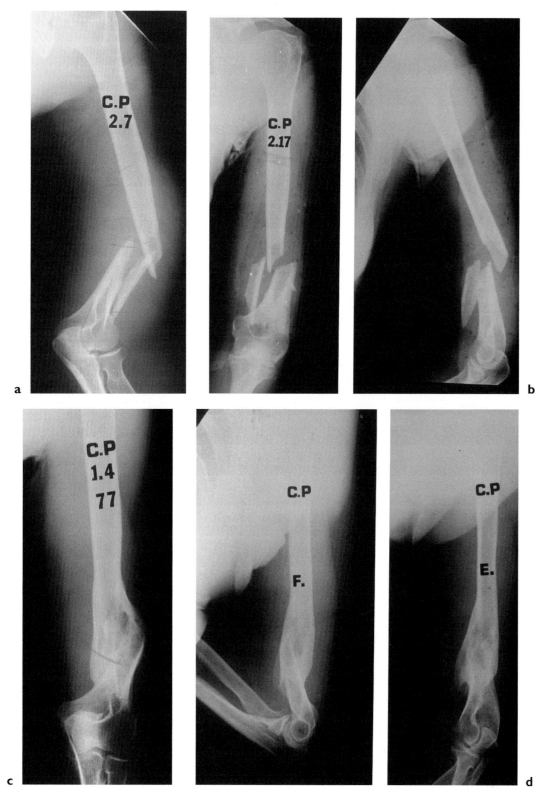

FIGURE 1.33. Comminuted fracture of the distal humerus is shown. Notice the severe varus angulation (**A**). The alignment of the fragments improved with the use of the functional brace (**B**). The fracture healed with significant angular deformity. The patient had not been instructed to prevent "leaning" on the elbow (**C**). The elbow regained full range of motion (**D**). *Continued.*

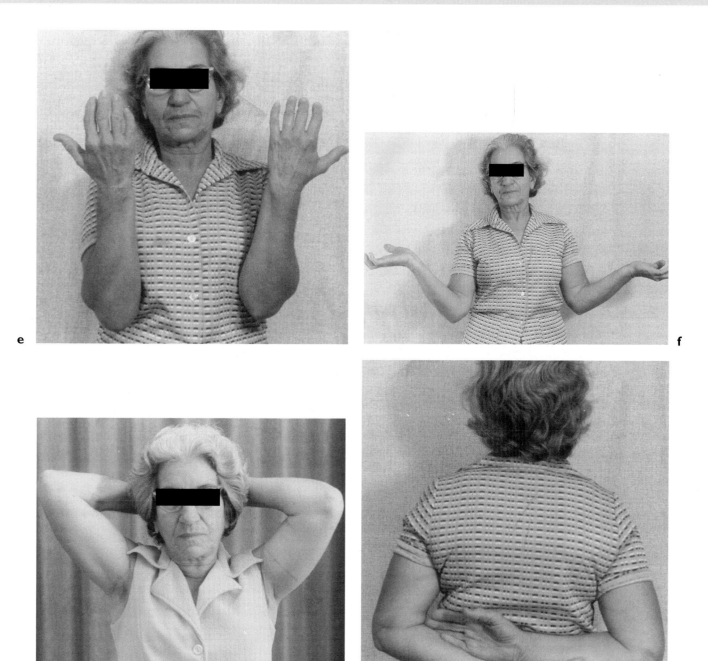

FIGURE 1.33. *Continued* The patient demonstrates the function of her elbow and shoulder joints (**E–H**).

COMPLICATIONS

LATE NERVE PALSY

Late onset of radial nerve palsy is rare but has been reported. It suggests entrapment of the nerve in the healing callus. The management of this complication is usually of a surgical nature. MRI studies should help in confirming the diagnosis of bony entrapment. Exploration of the nerve is necessary. Late palsy can also be seen following manipulation of a fracture, carried out in an attempt to improve fracture alignment.

MALALIGNMENT

We strongly discourage manipulation of diaphyseal humeral fractures and recommend unencumbered hanging of the arm at the side of the body. In the unlikely event the gradual increase of exercises fails to create an acceptable alignment, surgery is probably the treatment of choice.

Most angular deformities encountered with functional bracing of humeral shaft fractures are those of varus. This is particularly true for fractures below the middle third of the diaphysis (Figs. 1.19, 1.21, and 1.27). Proximal fractures usually develop valgus angulation (Fig. 1.29). The humeral diaphysis tolerates, functionally and cosmetically, angular deformities of degrees better than most other long bones. Arms with either large musculature or excessive adipose tissues camouflage deformity quite well.

Loss of the "carrying angle" of the elbow is very common, particularly in fractures of the distal third of the bone. Since women are more likely to have valgus elbows, a varus deformity of 15 to 20 degrees is difficult to recognize (Fig. 1.27).

Leaning on the elbow should be strongly discouraged as it produces angular deformities. This may occur during the initial period of cast immobilization but more likely after the application of the brace. This angular deformity is more likely to develop in transverse fractures (Fig. 1.34). Oblique or comminuted fractures experience during "weight bearing" shortening that recovers upon relaxation of the deforming force. This "piston motion" is osteogenic in nature.

Anteroposterior deformities can also develop and are more likely to be seen in transverse, nondisplaced fractures. A delay in reaching extension of the elbow may aggravate an anterior apex angulation. The "stiff elbow" that develops within the first 2 weeks creates abnormal stresses at the fracture site when the arm finally hangs over the side of the body. Patients with bilateral fractures, particularly if they had other associated injuries and are not capable of assuming the trunk's erect position, are more likely to develop such deformities (Fig. 1.35).

Most final angulation seen in humeral fractures managed by functional bracing is of a varus nature. The residual varus deformity implies a loss of the carrying angle of the elbow. We have not seen any impairment of function resulting from the loss of the few degrees of carrying angle the normal humerus has. Valgus deformity is rarely seen (Fig. 1.29).

Low-velocity gunshot-produced fractures are usually associated with some comminution—a factor that militates in favor of spontaneous healing. The associated degree of soft tissue pathology is usually mild. Therefore, the healing of these fractures takes place at a pace comparable with that of closed fractures. Oftentimes, the lateral displacement of the comminuted fragments enlarges the diameter of the bone at the level of the fracture. This enlarged diameter spontaneously decreases from the compression of the soft tissues by the functional sleeve and the gravity effect at the fracture site. The callus that forms under these circumstances is of a strong quality (Fig. 1.14).

DELAYED UNION AND NONUNION

It is not always easy to anticipate with precision when a fracture is likely to develop nonunion. In other long bone fractures, it is not uncommon to see fractures demonstrate no evidence of clinical or radiologic union for long periods of time and still observe eventual healing. The humerus seems to behave differently. A humeral diaphyseal fracture that demonstrates frank motion at the fracture site 1.5 months after the injury is not likely to unite spontaneously. Such motion is of a greater diagnostic significance than the absence of peripheral callus (5).

Fractures associated with peripheral nerve injury are the ones most likely to develop nonunion, particularly if the injured nerve affects the function of the flexor and extensor of the elbow. These fractures, as a rule, demonstrate initial axial separation between the fragments. This separation may be an ominous sign (Figs. 1.16 and 1.17). Axial distraction between fragments can also indicate major soft tissue damage that requires earlier active use of the surrounding musculature. Failure to see a rapid correction of the distraction often calls for surgical intervention.

SKIN PROBLEMS

Allergic reaction to the stockinet or plastic brace is extremely rare. Its occurrence calls for the local application of medications or discontinuation of the bracing technique. Since the brace can be easily removed and reapplied, daily hygienic measures, in most instances, prevent irritation or maceration of the skin.

REFRACTURE

The likelihood of refracture of long bones that heal with peripheral callus is extremely rare (Figs. 1.30 and 1.31). The strength of the bone at the level of the fracture is greater than before the fracture took place.

If a new injury occurs, the fracture will be located either above or below the original fracture. When a diaphyseal fracture is treated with methods that produce rigid immobilization of the fragments, the strength of the bone is significantly less than that in the remainder of the bone. Refractures under these circumstances are therefore more likely to occur.

LIMITATION OF MOTION

It is not unusual for diaphyseal humeral fractures treated with functional braces to heal with associated limitation of motion of the shoulder. The limitation is, in almost all instances, of a temporary nature. Continued use of the extremity usually brings about restoration of full range of motion.

Loss of external rotation is the most common limitation of motion. It is likely that the internal rotation position of the shoulder during the early stages of healing results in capsular contracture. The early conduct of pendulum exercises expedites recovery of motion.

Weakness of the surrounding arm musculature is inevitable, regardless of the method of treatment used. The early use of the extremity prevents signifi-

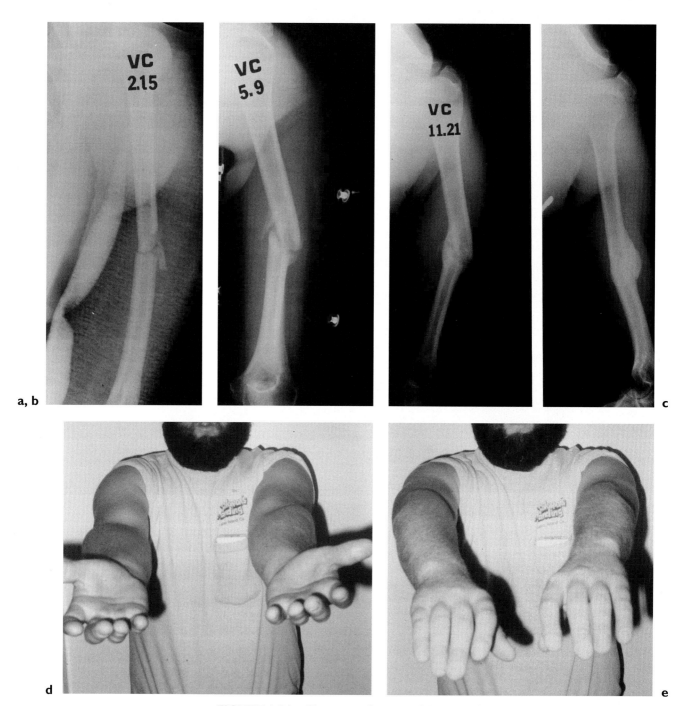

FIGURE 1.34. Transverse fracture of the humerus without displacement between the fragments is shown (**A**). Once the brace was applied and function was introduced, a varus deformity developed (**B**). The fracture healed with an angular varus deformity (**C**). However, the cosmetic appearance of the extremity remained acceptable due to the heavy musculature surrounding the humerus. Notice the loss of the carrying angle (**D–E**). *Continued.*

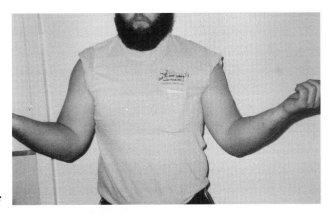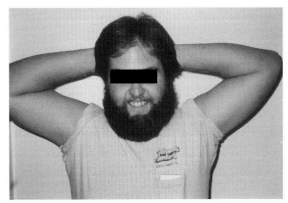

f   g

FIGURE 1.34. *Continued*   The range of motion of the elbow and shoulder was satisfactory.

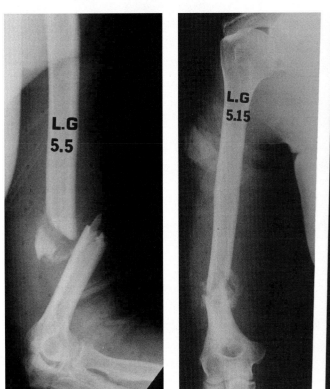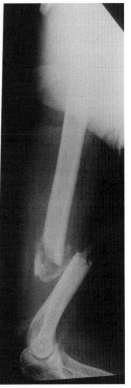

a   b

FIGURE 1.35.   Bilateral humeral fractures associated with other organ injuries are presented. The right humerus shows a fracture in its distal third with severe angulation (**A**). Healing progressed in the brace (**B**), and the fracture eventually healed but with a marked angular deformity (**C**). *Continued.*

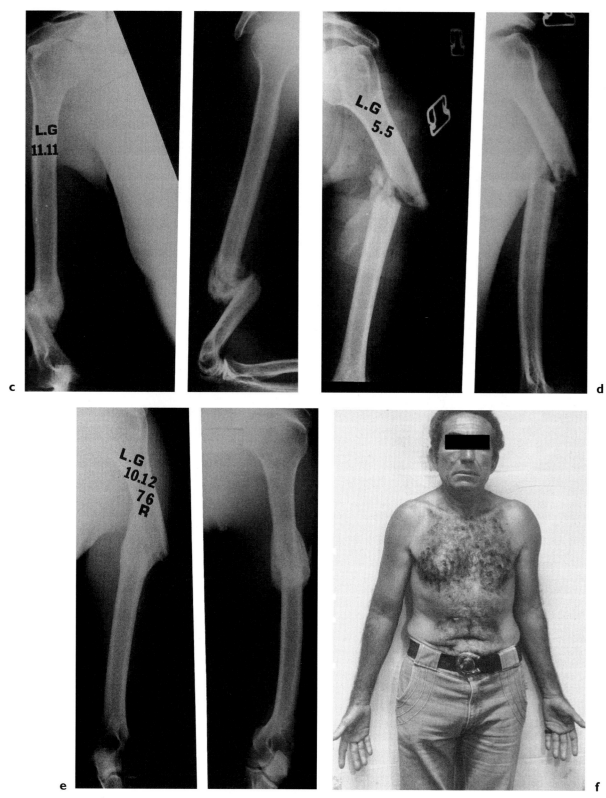

FIGURE 1.35. *Continued* The left humerus sustained a fracture at the junction of its proximal and middle thirds (**D**). The fracture healed with marked angular deformity (**E**). *Continued.*

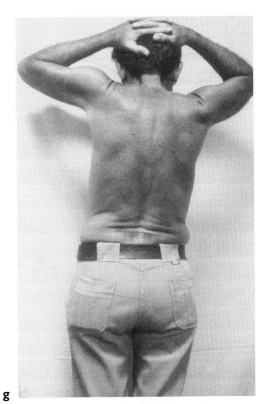

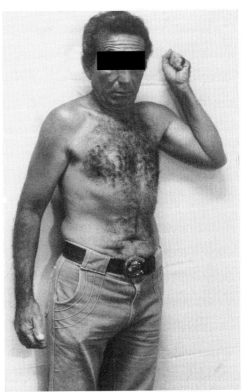

g

h

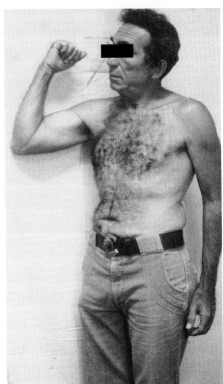

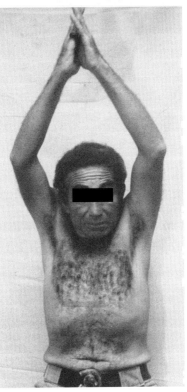

i

j

FIGURE 1.35. *Continued* The patient demonstrates the overall appearance of his upper extremities (**F**) as well as the range of motion of his elbows and shoulders (**F–J**).

cant weakness. It has been our experience that most patients can begin to combine passive exercises with active ones soon after the application of the brace. These exercises should apply to the flexors and extensor of the elbow.

The active contraction of these muscles not only prevents long-lasting muscle atrophy but assists in the correction of the frequently seen subluxation of the glenohumeral joint (Fig. 1.18). The contraction of the flexors and extensors of the elbow also assists in the correction of rotary deformities created by the parallel coiling of the fractured fragments and the surrounding musculature (Fig. 1.24).

RESULTS

Multiple reports have appeared in the orthopaedic literature dealing with functional bracing of diaphyseal humeral fractures. In this manual, we limit the presentation of results to those we obtained in our clinic and that we have reported in peer-reviewed journals (4–8,10).

One of our most recent reports was based on a series of 922 patients we treated in two different institutions: the University of Miami and the University of Southern California (8). However, of these 922 patients, only 620 (67%) were available for complete clinical and radiographic evaluation. Four hundred sixty-five (75%) of the fractures were closed, and 155 (25%) were open.

Healing took place at an average of 11.5 weeks (range 5 to 22 weeks). The 465 closed fractures healed at a median of 9.5 weeks (range 5 to 19 weeks) and the 155 open fractures at a mean of 14 weeks (range 8 to 22 weeks).

Nerve function did not return in 1 of the 67 patients who had radial nerve palsy. The 12 patients who had an inferior subluxation of the glenohumeral joint demonstrated spontaneous correction of the subluxation. Four (<1%) of the patients had a refracture between the second and eighth week after removal of the brace. Angular deformities were measured in 565 (91%) patients. The 101 transverse fractures healed with an average of 9 degrees of varus angulation, the 149 oblique fractures with an average of 4 degrees, and the 364 comminuted fractures with an average of 8 degrees. Nine patients (6%) who had an open fracture and seven (<2%) who had a closed fracture had a nonunion.

In 87% of the 565 patients for whom anteroposterior radiographs were available, the fracture healed in <16 degrees of varus angulation. In 81% of the 546 for whom lateral radiographs wee available, it healed in <16 degrees of anterior angulation.

At the time of brace removal, 98% of the patients had limitation of shoulder motion of ≤25 degrees. It was anticipated that continued use of the extremity would result in a further improvement in motion.

The cost of care of humeral shaft fractures by surgical and nonsurgical means has been studied and found to be much greater when surgery is performed.

BASIC GUIDELINES FOR PHYSICIANS

DIAPHYSEAL HUMERAL FRACTURES

1. **Indications for functional braces:** Functional braces are indicated for most isolated closed diaphyseal fractures of the humeral diaphysis as well as open fractures with only a moderate degree of soft tissue damage.

2. **Relative contraindications:** Functional braces are contraindicated for fractures with major soft tissue pathology. These fractures, when accompanied with peripheral nerve palsy, do poorly when treated by nonsurgical means. Closed or open fractures that demonstrate distal distraction between the fragments are likely to develop nonunion if treated by closed means. Braces are also contraindicated in most patients with bilateral humeral fractures and those with multiple organ injuries or with multiple fractures.

3. **How high or low in the diaphysis the fracture can be:** Proximal metaphyseal fractures require other modalities of care, that is, sling or internal or external fixation. Fractures of the humeral head are also treated with either slings, internal fixation, or prosthetic replacement. It is not necessary for the brace to fully cover the fracture site. Compression of the surrounding tissues is the essential prerequisite.

4. **When to brace:** It is best to wait a minimum of 1 week before the application of the brace. Swelling of the distal extremity and excessive pain are likely to develop when the brace is applied too early. A long arm cast is probably the best means to initially stabilize diaphyseal humeral fractures.

5. **Exercises to be performed:** Pendulum exercises must begin as soon as possible. As soon as the brace is applied, the exercises continue with the arm supported in a collar and cuff. Within a few days, the passive exercises are combined with assistive active exercises. Efforts should be made to regain elbow extension during the first 2 weeks after brace application. Once full extension is reached, passive circumduction exercises can be carried out without the need for the sling, which can be discontinued during the day but used during recumbency.

6. **How to adjust the brace and when to remove it temporarily:** The straps of the brace must be frequently tightened. If the brace slips distally, it should be brought back to the appropriate level and then tightened.

7. **Activities to be avoided:** Active flexion or elevation of the shoulder should not be permitted before radiologic demonstration of good stabilizing callus. These exercises might create angular deformities. Leaning on the elbow should also be avoided to lessen the likelihood of similar deformities. Transverse fractures experience the greatest angular deformities.

8. **When the brace can be permanently discontinued:** Once solid union of the fracture has been documented clinically and radiographically, the brace can be permanently discontinued. A residual limitation of shoulder motion, particularly external rotation, will remain for a period of time. Rarely is permanent limitation of motion observed, except in elderly patients.

9. **The severity of an angular deformity that can be accepted:** Most major deformities can be prevented by allowing dependency of the extremity and compression of the tissues. The humeral diaphysis tolerates angular deformities that other long bones do not tolerate. Fifteen degrees of varus angulation is almost always impossible to detect.

BASIC GUIDELINES FOR PATIENTS

DIAPHYSEAL HUMERAL FRACTURES

1. **Activities:** The plastic brace is usually applied within the first 2 weeks after the injury, following removal of the initial cast. A sling is also used to support the broken arm. Pendulum exercises should begin as soon as possible to prevent permanent limitation of motion of the shoulder. The exercises, if gently performed, should not produce pain, and the discomfort should gradually disappear.

   After a few days, the arm may be temporarily removed from the sling, using the normal hand, and gradual attempts begun to flex and extend the elbow. If done several times, full extension of the elbow is achieved within 1 to 2 weeks. When the elbow reaches full extension, the sling can be discontinued during the day but should be kept in place while lying down. The pendulum exercises continue with the elbow in full extension. If pain accompanies the normal swing of the arm, the sling should be reapplied until the symptoms completely disappear.

2. **Adjusting the brace:** The brace must compress the arm snugly at all times. The snug appliance provides greater comfort. As the swelling decreases, the brace gets loose and slips distally toward the elbow. This should be corrected as it happens, by further loosening the Velcro straps and bringing the brace upward to its original position. After a few days, the need to adjust the brace decreases as the swelling decreases.

3. **Prohibitions:** Patients wearing a brace should not try to elevate the arm either forward or laterally because the weight of the limb can angulate the broken bone. This type of exercise may be carried out only after radiographs have shown progressive healing and there is no longer pain at the fracture site. Leaning on the elbow may result in permanent deformities. The arm should hang to the side of the body at all times.

4. **Loosening the brace for hygienic purposes:** Temporary loosening of the brace for hygienic purposes may be done as often as desired. The Velcro straps should be firmly tightened upon completion of the task.

5. **Permanent removal of the brace:** The brace should not be discontinued until radiographs have confirmed solid healing of the fracture. Most fractures heal within 3 to 4 months.

6. **Expectations:** Upon removal of the brace, most patients notice limitation of shoulder motion in certain directions. Continued use of the shoulder and the resumption of activities of daily living usually result in a resolution of the limitation of motion. Elderly people are more likely to suffer prolonged periods of disability. The broken humerus usually heals with a few degrees of angulation. In most instances, the deformity is not noticed and is not associated with limitation of function. Appropriate use of the brace is rarely accompanied with visible deformities.

REFERENCES

1. Balfour GW, Mooney V, Ashby ME. Diaphyseal fractures of the humerus treated with a ready-made fracture brace. *J Bone Joint Surg (Am)* 1982;64:11.

2. McMaster WC, Tivnon MC, Waugh TR. Cast brace for the upper extremity. *Clin Orthop* 1975;109:126.

3. Naver L, Aalberg JR. Humeral shaft fractures treated with a ready-made fracture brace. *Arch Orthop Trauma Surg* 1986;106:20.

4. Sarmiento A, Horowitch A, Aboulafia A, et al. Functional bracing of comminuted extra-articular fractures of the distal third of the humerus. *J Bone Joint Surg (Br)* 1990;72:283.

5. Sarmiento A, Kinman PB, Galvin EG, et al. Functional bracing of fractures of the shaft of the humerus. *J Bone Joint Surg (Am)* 1977;59:596.

6. Sarmiento A, Latta LL. *Closed functional treatment of fractures*. Berlin: Springer-Verlag, 1981.

7. Sarmiento A, Latta LL. *Functional fracture bracing*. Heidelberg: Springer-Verlag, 1995.

8. Sarmiento A, Latta LL, Zych GA, et al. Functional bracing of humeral shaft fractures. *J Bone Joint Surg (Am)* 1999;82:478–486.

9. Sarmiento A, Waddell J, Latta LL. Diaphyseal humeral fractures: treatment options. *J Bone Joint Surg* 2001;83-A:1566–1579.

10. Sarmiento A, Watson T. Functional bracing of diaphyseal humeral fractures and operative management of humeral shaft fractures. In: *Fractures: diagnosis and treatment*. New York: McGraw-Hill, 2000:225–242.

11. Wasmer G, Worsdorfer O. Functional management of humeral shaft fractures with Sarmiento cast bracing. *Unfallheilkunde* 1984;87:309.

12. Zagorski JB, Latta LL, Zych GA, et al. Diaphyseal fractures of the humerus—treatment with prefabricated braces. *J Bone Joint Surg (Am)* 1988;70:607.

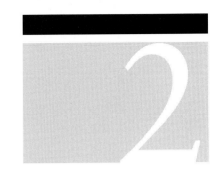

Functional Bracing of Diaphyseal Ulnar Fractures

Rationale

Indications and Contraindications

Acute Management

    Closed Fractures

    Open Fractures

Brace Application and Function

Patient Instructions

Brace Removal and Follow-Up

Expected Outcome

Managing Complications

    Synostosis

    Malalignment

    Delayed Union and Nonunion

    Skin Problems

    Refracture

    Limitation of Motion and Loss of Strength

Application of Functional Brace

    Prefabricated Brace

    Brace Application

    Postbracing Management and Maintenance

Results

Basic Guidelines for Physicians

Basic Guidelines for Patients

References

RATIONALE

Plating of isolated ulnar fractures is a popular method of treatment, and the overall reported results are mixed. Postoperative infection is low, and nonunion and implant failure do not occur with great frequency. However, refracture is not uncommon, and the cost of surgical treatment remains higher (5).

The popularity of surgical plating of isolated ulnar fractures came as a result of observing that nonunion was occasionally encountered when the limb was immobilized in casts that extended from the head of the metacarpals to above the elbow. Such a long cast had been used in accommodation to the long-held premise that joints above and below a fracture required immobilization. Today, such practice has been proved flawed, and evidence that freedom of motion of joints and physiologically induced motion at the fracture site are beneficial has replaced that concept (3,4). Watson Jones, whose influence in the practice of orthopaedics a half century ago was significant, stated that the high incidence of nonunion in ulnar fractures treated with long arm casts was due to the fact that the cast did not provide the degree of immobilization required for healing to occur (6). The fact that the union rate with functional "sleeves," which do not immobilize either the elbow or the wrist, is only about 2 percent strongly suggests that if nonunion is common with long arm casts, it is because the casts immobilize too much, rather than not enough (1).

The high rate of success with functional bracing of isolated ulnar fractures makes it difficult to justify routine plating of these fractures. There are, however, instances when open surgery is the treatment of choice.

The fact that the ulna is firmly attached to the radius makes major angular and rotary deformities in isolated ulnar fractures extremely rare. The intact radius prevents shortening of the fractured ulna, and the strong interosseous membrane precludes major displacement of the fragments. The significant stability of the proximal and distal radioulnar joints prevents rotary deformities.

INDICATIONS AND CONTRAINDICATIONS

Most isolated ulnar fractures are the result of a direct blow over the forearm, and in most instances, the fracture is of a closed type. When a fracture of the ulnar diaphysis occurs after a fall on the outstretched hand, an associated dislocation of the radial head is almost always present. This condition, known as a Monteggia fracture, is a clear indication for surgical intervention due to the difficulties encountered in maintaining a manually achieved reduction of the joint. The above observations suggest that the majority of isolated ulnar fractures can be successfully treated with functional braces that permit early use of the extremity, without the need for the prevention of pronosupination of the forearm and flexion and extension of the elbow and wrist.

Low-grade open fractures can also be treated in this manner after appropriate debridement of the injured soft tissues. More severe open fractures associated with major soft tissue damage may require stabilization with external fixators until the condition of the area is satisfactory and free of infection. At that point, internal fixation and bone grafting may be indicated. Plating under these circumstances may be risky.

ACUTE MANAGEMENT

CLOSED FRACTURES

To provide relief from the acute pain that accompanies all fractures, we prefer to stabilize the arm in an above-the-elbow cast that holds the elbow in a position of 90 degrees of flexion and the forearm in a relaxed attitude of supination. The position of relaxed supination is more likely to place the fragments in the most anatomical alignment and separate the two bones to the maximum degree. In addition, it helps in restoring earlier pronosupination of the forearm, owing to the fact that routine daily activities call for the use of pronation more frequently than supination. In other words, patients, through necessity, pronate their forearm and regain the initially lost motion. In the event that a permanent loss of motion of the forearm occurs, it is best to lose the last few degrees of pronation rather than supination. The shoulder girdle, through an inconspicuous motion of flexion, internal rotation, and abduction, compensates for that loss. A comparable inconspicuous mechanism for the loss of supination does not exist. This is the mechanism used by upper extremity amputees to compensate for the absence of forearm pronosupination.

The initial long arm cast is not always necessary. If the energy that produces the fracture is moderate and the accompanying pain and swelling are not significant, a below-the-elbow cast or splint may suffice. In those instances, the functional brace can be applied initially (5,7,8).

When a cast or splint is used initially, it does not need to be held in place for >1 week. Most patients, at that time, experience only minimal to moderate discomfort. Those who use their fingers and wrist from the very outset are more likely to get rid of pain sooner. This is particularly important to keep in mind when dealing with bilateral fractures.

OPEN FRACTURES

Low-energy-produced open fractures rarely demonstrate significant displacement between the fracture fragments. The intact radius and interosseous membrane prevent major displacement. In open fractures resulting from high-energy injuries and associated with major soft tissue damage, the displacement between the fragments may be significant owing to damage to the stabilizing interosseous membrane. These fractures require appropriate debridement of the wound and, not infrequently, stabilization with plates or external fixators. Less severe fractures may be managed with functional braces as soon as the wounds begin to show healthy signs of healing. The presence of an open wound does not preclude the use of braces as they are removable and permit cleansing of the wound and frequent dressing changes.

BRACE APPLICATION AND FUNCTION

The initial above-the-elbow cast may be removed at the end of the first week. The brace is then applied. A sling or collar and cuff is also applied to eliminate the pain that the dependent arm is likely to produce.

The brace ("sleeve") permits unencumbered use of the arm because it does not extend over the elbow or wrist (Fig. 2.1). It simply limits pronosupination. The brace must be adjustable in order to effectively compress the soft tissues and in that manner provide comfort.

PATIENT INSTRUCTIONS

Patients are encouraged to use the extremity to the maximum degree allowed by pain. In most instances, the pain present at the time of application of the brace is only moderate. It is our opinion that the early introduction of function results in a more rapid disappearance of acute symptoms and faster healing.

The brace should be adjusted on a frequent basis during the first few days to maintain the desirable compression of the soft tissues and to prevent the distal displacement of the sleeve over the wrist. The brace may be removed for hygienic purposes as often as necessary and the collar and cuff permanently discontinued as soon as the symptoms subside.

Flexion and extension of the elbow are rapidly regained. Pronation and supination require a longer period of time because such motions are more painful (Fig. 2.2). In a few instances, we have treated patients with functional braces who had sustained bilateral isolated ulnar fractures. Their recovery was relatively rapid and uneventful.

BRACE REMOVAL AND FOLLOW-UP

The brace is permanently discontinued as soon as the symptoms subside. We do not believe the brace is necessary after that time, even if the radiologically detected healing is not complete. For reasons not fully understood by us, there are times when bony callus does not develop rapidly, suggesting the possibility of a possible nonunion. Continued use of the extremity eventually produces the radiologically pleasing bony callus in most instances (Fig. 2.3).

EXPECTED OUTCOME

At the time of completion of healing, there is usually full range of motion of the elbow. The motion of the wrist may be slightly limited for an additional few weeks, particularly when the fracture is located close to the wrist joint. A mild permanent loss of pronation and supination is found in a small percentage of patients, particularly in those with fractures located in the proximal third of the bone. This limitation of motion is usually compensated inconspicuously through shoulder rotation. The overall functional results are most gratifying.

MANAGING COMPLICATIONS

We are not aware of any complications that can be directly traced to the brace other than possible allergic reaction to the stockinet or to the plastic material of the appliance. Increase of angulation at the fracture site has not been reported. The intrinsic stability of the fracture provided by the interosseous membrane ensures that the original displacement will remain unchanged. Nonunion and infection are unrelated to the bracing treatment.

SYNOSTOSIS

Synostosis is extremely rare when isolated ulnar fractures are treated with functional braces. Perhaps the early introduction of function prevents the building of a bridge between the two bones. Synostosis is more common after plate fixation. Fractures associated with head injuries are known to develop heterotopic bone. We had the opportunity to observe three such instances of synostosis after an isolated ulnar fracture treated with a functional brace. This complication requires surgical excision of the bony bridge. The prognosis is not always good as a residual limitation of motion is usually identified.

MALALIGNMENT

As most fractures occur from a direct blow over the forearm, the degree of displacement of the fragments is usually minor (Fig. 2.4). The associated damage of the interosseous membrane is also minimal. This explains the mild displacement. The direction of the blow obviously dictates the displacement of the fragments, which in most instances is toward the intact radius (Figs. 2.5 to 2.7). It is in this instance that damage of the interosseous membrane is the mildest. When the displacement of the fragments is either dorsal or volar, the soft tissue damage is greater. Nonetheless, shortening does not take place on account of the intact radius.

DELAYED UNION AND NONUNION

Most isolated ulnar fractures demonstrate radiologic union within 2 to 2.5 months. Most demonstrate large peripheral callus, indicating the beneficial effect of motion at the fracture site. There are instances, however, when a gap between the fragments remains present for a longer period of time, suggesting a delayed union or a nonunion (Fig. 2.7). If the associated symptoms are minimal or nonexistent, skillful neglect is the most appropriate approach. Almost without exception, radiologic healing eventually becomes apparent. Failure to achieve painless bony union calls for surgery and possibly a grafting procedure.

SKIN PROBLEMS

Allergic reactions to the stockinet of plastic material are rare. Poor hygiene is the most likely cause of skin irritation. The frequent removal of the brace and washing of the arm and hand, which is possible and recommended from the very outset, prevent skin problems. If present, skin problems are probably due to excessive perspiration and a reaction to heat.

REFRACTURE

Diaphyseal fractures treated with functional braces usually heal with peripheral callus. Under those circumstances, the likelihood of refracture is minimal. The new bone at the level of the fracture is stronger than before the fracture (5). The thinning of the bony cortices, frequently seen under plates, does not occur. If a new fracture were to occur, its management would not differ from the original one.

LIMITATION OF MOTION AND LOSS OF STRENGTH

It is logical to expect a temporary weakness of grip in all patients who sustain diaphyseal ulnar fractures. However, because the period of inactivity is relatively short, the resulting muscular weakness is mild and the recovery thereof is rapid. The same applies to the residual limitation of motion. Many patients demonstrate a mild loss of pronation of the forearm, but inconspicuous compensation occurs from mild flexion, abduction, and internal rotation of the shoulder. This mechanism is similar to that used by below-the-elbow amputees

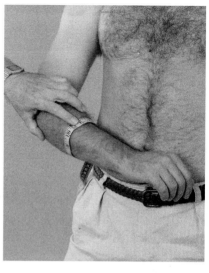
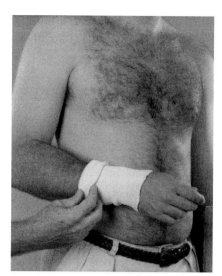

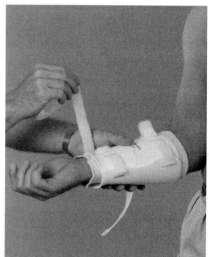
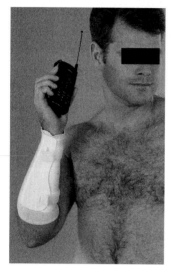

a, b

c, d

FIGURE 2.1. The various steps taken for the application of the functional brace are illustrated. The girth of the forearm is measured to select the appropriate size of the brace (**A**). A stockinet is rolled over the forearm, which is held in a relaxed attitude of supination (**B**). The brace is fastened with Velcro straps (**C**). The brace was designed to compress soft tissues in an anteroposterior direction to best separate the radius from the ulna (**D**).

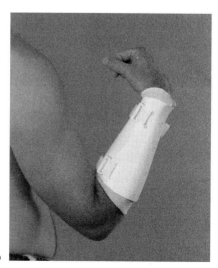
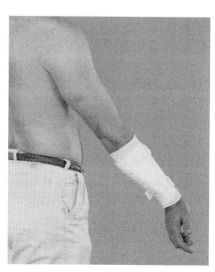

a, b

FIGURE 2.2. After a few days, the patient wearing the functional brace should be able to fully flex and extend the elbow joint (**A and B**) as well as pronate and supinate the forearm (**C and D**). *Continued.*

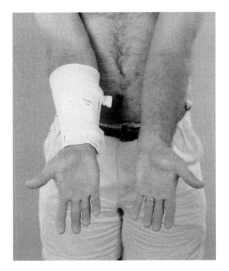
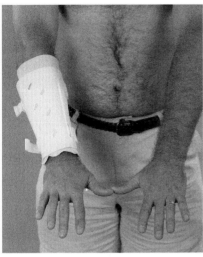

FIGURE 2.2. *Continued*   **c, d**

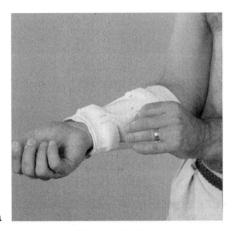
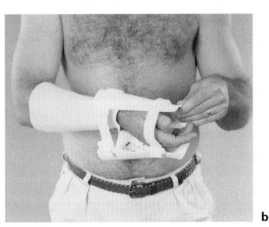

a   b

FIGURE 2.3.   The brace is easily removed for hygienic purposes by releasing the Velcro straps (**A**) and then slipping the "sleeve" distally over the wrist and hand (**B**).

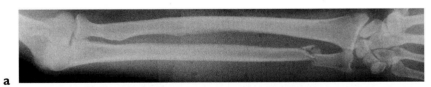

a

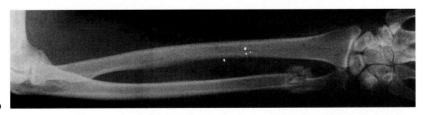

b

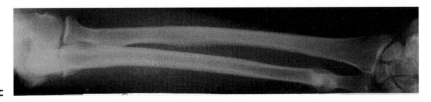

c

FIGURE 2.4. Composite of radiographs of a fracture of the distal end of the ulna illustrates the initial mild displacement between the fragments (**A**), the early evidence of peripheral callus 4 weeks after the initial insult (**B**), and the solidly united fracture 3 months after injury (**C**).

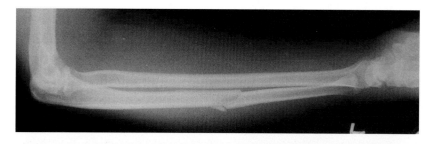

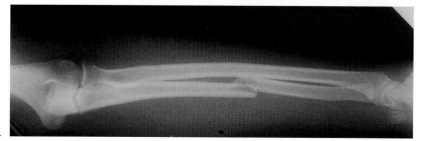

a

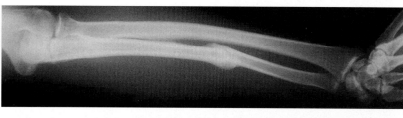

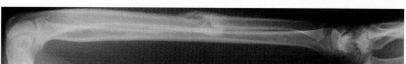

b

FIGURE 2.5. Anteroposterior and lateral radiographs of isolated closed fracture in the middle third of the ulna are presented (**A**). Radiographs obtained after completion of union demonstrate the inconsequential mild lateral angular deformity at the fracture site (**B**). The patient demonstrates the functional range of pronosupination at the time of removal of the brace (**C and D**).

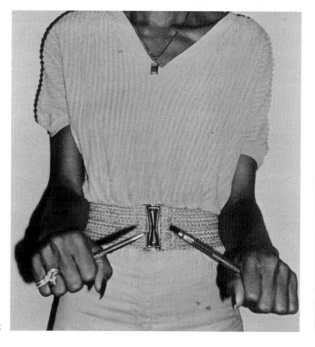

c

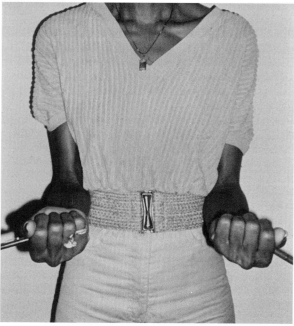

d

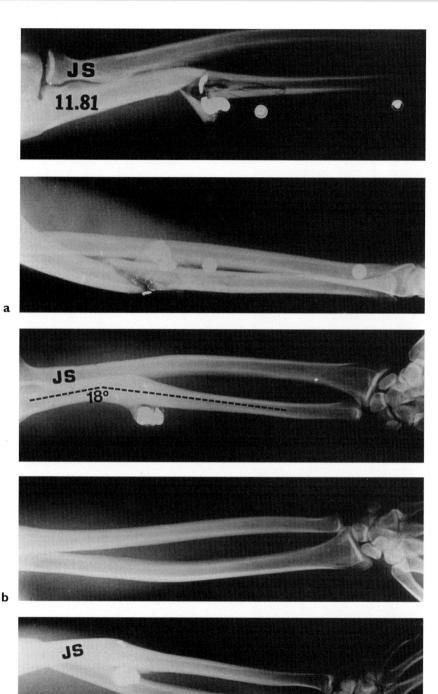

FIGURE 2.6. Comminuted fracture of the ulna at the junction of the proximal and middle third of the ulna was the result of a gunshot injury (**A**). Radiographs of both forearms in supination after completion of healing demonstrate the similar range of supination in both forearms (**B**). Radiographs of both forearms in pronation demonstrate the mild limitation of pronation in the fractured extremity (**C**). This degree of limitation of pronation is inconspicuously compensated by shoulder rotation.

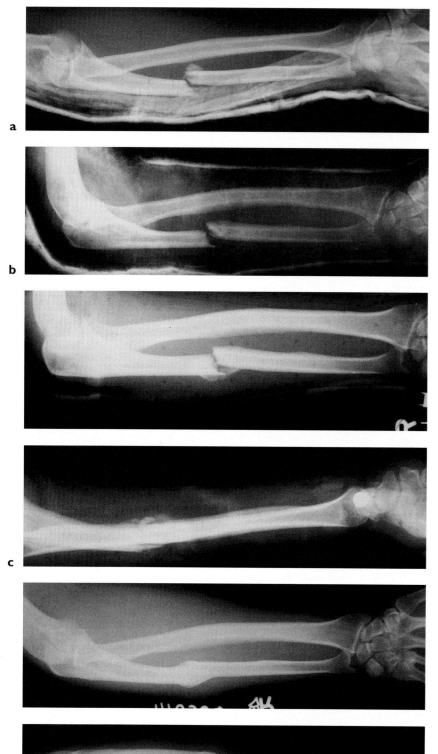

FIGURE 2.7. Initial radiograph of slightly oblique isolated fracture of the ulna demonstrates mild angular deformity (**A**) apparent in the initial above-the-elbow cast (**B**). Anteroposterior and lateral radiographs obtained through the functional brace depict early healing with peripheral callus (**C**). Radiographs illustrate solid union of the fracture. A mild inconsequential angular deformity persisted (**D**).

who pronate the terminal device in a comparable manner. The limitation of pronation detected at the time the brace is permanently discontinued improves with return to normal activities.

APPLICATION OF FUNCTIONAL BRACE

PREFABRICATED BRACE

The ulnar fracture brace, or "sleeve," must be adjustable to make possible its frequent removal and reapplication for hygienic purposes and to ensure the maintenance of its desirable snugness against the soft tissues. Velcro straps are best for this purpose. Circular casts that cannot be adjusted slip distally as swelling subsides and atrophy of the musculature takes place. The brace should be short enough to make possible free motion of the wrist and elbow, regardless of the location of the fracture (Fig. 2.1). Obviously, rigid immobilization of fragments is not necessary. What the brace accomplishes is probably nothing more than provision of comfort and protection to the arm from inadvertent forceful contact with hard objects.

BRACE APPLICATION

It is preferable to use cotton stockinet under the brace that extends from just above the wrist to just below the elbow. It can be washed and replaced as often as necessary. The patient's forearm should be held in a relaxed attitude of supination during the application of the brace. The snugness of the brace should not be too great because distal swelling can occur as a result of the tourniquet-like effect of the brace.

The ulnar brace, as in the case of the humerus and tibia, can be custommade or prefabricated. It can be made of casting material or of plastics.

POSTBRACING MANAGEMENT AND MAINTENANCE

Patients should avoid prolonged dependency of the injured extremity because of the likely possibility of distal edema developing. Frequent tightening of the fist and wrist-active exercises assist in the prevention and correction of this problem.

The patient can temporarily remove the brace to carry out active pronosupination of the forearm when the degree of discomfort permits it. Most patients seem to be able to do so after 1 week of wearing the brace. Washing of the forearm can be done as often as desired.

RESULTS

The management of isolated diaphyseal ulnar fractures with functional bracing has been frequently discussed in the orthopaedic literature. In this manual, we limit the discussion of results to those we have ourselves reported in peer-reviewed orthopaedic journals (2,4,5,7,8).

Our most recent published report is based on a combined project between two major teaching institutions: the University of Miami and the University of Southern California (5). This report is based on 444 patients treated with prefabricated ulnar braces. From this group, only 287 (65%) were available to complete follow-up. A large percentage of patients failed to return to medical follow-up once the symptoms disappeared.

Ninety-nine percent of the fractures healed spontaneously. Shortening of the ulna averaged 1.1 mm. This is understandable in view of the fact that the radius was intact in all instances and those fractured ulnas with associated radial dislocation were not treated with functional braces.

Final radial angulation averaged 5 degrees (range 0 to 18 degrees). Dorsal angulation averaged 5 degrees (range 0 to 20 degrees).

Average loss of pronation was greatest in fractures of the proximal third of the ulna, averaging 12 degrees. Fractures of the middle third of the ulna had a loss of pronation of 10 degrees (range 0 to 45 degrees) and a loss of supination of 2 degrees. Fractures of the distal third averaged a loss of 5 degrees of pronation.

Three patients (1%) with open fractures developed a synostosis between the radius and the ulna, eliminating all pronation and supination. These patients had concomitant head injuries.

The cost of care of isolated ulnar fractures with functional braces was compared with the cost of care of similar fractures treated with plate fixation. The cost of acute care with functional bracing was $1,529. The cost of plate fixation was $8,671. These data do not include possible subsequent hospitalizations and surgery such as plate removal, infection, etc (5).

BASIC GUIDELINES FOR PHYSICIANS

ISOLATED ULNAR FRACTURES

1. **Indications:** Most closed and low-grade open isolated ulnar fractures may be treated with functional braces. As most of these fractures are the result of a direct blow over the extremity and the radius is intact, shortening is not present. For the same reasons, severe angular deformities are very rare.

2. **Contraindications:** (a) Ulnar fractures associated with dislocation of the radiocapitellar joint should not be braced. Surgical stabilization is the treatment of choice. (b) Open fractures, the result of severe injuries that demonstrate marked displacement between the fragments, suggesting extensive soft tissue pathology, should not braced. (c) Bracing is contraindicated in fractures of the proximal third with major angulation.

3. **When to brace:** Most isolated ulnar fractures may be braced at approximately 1 week after the initial injury. If pain and swelling are minimal, the brace may be applied earlier.

4. **Activities:** The brace does not immobilize the elbow or wrist joint. The mild pain that necessarily accompanies all fractures limits the degree of activities in which the patient may indulge. Pronation and supination are the motions most likely to be temporarily limited.

5. **Removal of brace for hygienic purposes:** The brace should be snugly applied. The snugness brings about greater comfort. It may be temporarily loosened at any time. It is desirable to attempt gradual increase of forearm rotation.

6. **When to permanently discontinue the brace:** The brace may be permanently discontinued when radiographs demonstrate bridging callus. Often, radiologically visible bridging requires a long time to appear. If symptoms are absent, the brace may be discontinued.

7. **Expectations:** Most patients experience healing of their isolated ulnar fractures with minimal or no limitation of motion of the forearm. As the initial cast and subsequent brace hold the forearm in a relaxed attitude of supination, restoration of full pronation is delayed. Such temporary loss of pronation is easily and inconspicuously compensated for with shoulder rotation. The average healing time is around 2 to 2.5 months.

BASIC GUIDELINES FOR PATIENTS

ISOLATED ULNAR FRACTURES

1. **Activities:** After the application of the brace, patients should be able to carry out any activities. The degree of discomfort at the fracture site should be the guide. Some discomfort at the fracture site is expected to be present for several days, but it should decrease as activity increases. The brace should be held snugly over the forearm to minimize discomfort. Active use of the arm seems to enhance healing.

2. **When to loosen the brace for hygienic purposes:** The brace may be loosened for hygienic purposes as often as desired. When the brace is loosened, gentle attempts to rotate the forearm should be made. Pain should dictate the degree of excursion.

3. **When to remove the brace permanently:** The brace may be removed permanently when radiographs demonstrate adequate healing of the fracture or there is complete absence of symptoms with only partial radiographic healing.

4. **Expectations:** Most fractured ulnas heal within 3 months. A mild permanent limitation of motion of forearm rotation may be seen. When present, it is likely to be of only a few degrees, which usually goes unnoticed as it is easily compensated by rotation of the shoulder. This loss of pronosupination rarely precludes the conduct of normal activities. If the fracture was a severe one and was associated with major skin damage, the likelihood of permanent limitation of motion is greater. Fractures located in the proximal third of the ulna are more likely to experience greater limitation of motion.

REFERENCES

1. Pollock FH, Pankovich AM, Prieto JJ, et al. The isolated fracture of the ulnar shaft—treatment without immobilization. *J Bone Joint Surg (Am)* 1983;65:339.
2. Sarmiento A, Kinman PB, Murphy RB, et al. Treatment of ulnar fractures by functional bracing. *J Bone Joint Surg (Am)* 1976;58:1104.
3. Sarmiento A, Latta LL. Functional fracture bracing. *J Am Acad Orthop Surg* 1999;7: 66–78.
4. Sarmiento A, Latta LL, Tarr RR. Principles of fracture healing—part II: the effect of function on fracture healing and stability. In: *AAOS instructional course lectures, 23.* St. Louis: Mosby, 1984.
5. Sarmiento A, Latta L, Zych G, et al. Functional bracing of isolated ulnar fractures. *J Orthop Trauma* 1996;12:420–424.
6. Watson-Jones R. *Fractures and other bone and joint injuries.* Baltimore: Williams & Wilkins, 1941.
7. Zagorski JB, Zych GA, Latta LL, et al. Modern concepts in functional fracture bracing—upper limb. In: *AAOS instructional course lectures, 26.* Chicago: American Association of Orthopaedic Surgeons, 1987.
8. Zych GA, Zagorski JB, Latta LL. Treatment of isolated ulnar fractures with prefabricated fracture braces. *Clin Orthop* 1987;219:1944.

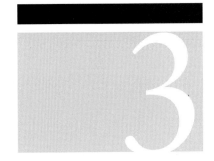

Functional Bracing of Diaphyseal Tibial Fractures

Rationale

Indications and Contraindications

Acute Management

    Closed Fractures

    Open Fractures

Manipulation

Initial Immobilization

Patient Instructions

Follow-Up

Expected Outcome

Managing Complications

    Late Nerve Palsy

    Malalignment and Shortening

    Delayed Union and Nonunion

Initial Stabilization

Below-the-Knee Functional Cast

Application of Functional Brace

    Custom-Made Brace

    Thermoplastic Custom-Made Brace

    Prefabricated Brace

Results

Basic Guidelines for Physicians

Basic Guidelines for Patients

References

RATIONALE

As in the case of other diaphyseal fractures, the philosophy of functional bracing of diaphyseal tibial fractures is predicated on the principle that physiologically induced motion at the fracture site is conducive to osteogenesis and therefore immobilization of adjacent joints and rigid fixation of fragments are detrimental to fracture healing.

We have documented that closed diaphyseal tibial fractures experience, at the time of the injury, the maximum amount of shortening and that the subsequent introduction of graduated weight bearing or muscle function does not produce additional shortening (31,37–40) (see Figs. I.1 to I.4). The degree of soft tissue detachment from the bone determines the initial shortening. This explains why, in general, open and high-energy-produced fractures demonstrate greater shortening than closed and low-energy-produced fractures.

Neither a cast nor a brace prevents shortening of a limb with a closed fracture if the fracture is axially unstable, that is, oblique, comminuted, and subjected to gradual weight-bearing or muscular activities. Axially unstable fractures, which are subjected to traction to regain length, experience a recurrence of shortening to the initial degree, particularly if subjected to weight-bearing stresses (see Fig. I.1).

Braces do not prevent shortening. They simply stabilize fragments against angular forces. This is accomplished through a hydraulic mechanism provided by the water-rich soft tissues surrounding the fractured bones (34,37).

Transverse fractures that do not displace originally or those that are manipulated and reduced obviously do not shorten (Figs. 3.2 and 3.3). Properly used casts or braces simply prevent angular deformities.

In axially unstable fractures, that is, oblique, spiral, and comminuted, weight bearing and/or active motion of the ankle produce elastic motions at the fracture site. The extremity shortens during weight bearing and/or muscle contractions but returns to the initial shortening during the swing phase of gait and during rest. These motions have a major beneficial effect, documented by findings in experimental animals when oblique fractures form a stronger callus than the transverse, stable transverse ones (29,31). Clinical experiences have supported the laboratory findings.

If the technology is available, the surgeon is trained in its use, and the infrastructure of the health care facility is appropriate, it is best to use intramedullary nailing or external fixation in the management of tibial diaphysis fractures that experience excessive and unacceptable initial shortening. The same applies to closed fractures with severe angular deformities that cannot be corrected by manual techniques.

Most closed diaphyseal fractures of the tibia experience <12 mm of initial shortening (Figs. 3.1 and 3.4). This means that most closed tibial fractures heal with <1 cm of shortening. It is our opinion this 10 mm of shortening is acceptable under all circumstances as it does not produce a limp or have adverse sequelae on the adjacent joints. Tall people seem to tolerate well as much as 1.5 cm of shortening without a resulting limp.

There are times when the acceptance of 1.5 cm is appropriate. The patient's advanced age, associated injuries, or general condition can fully justify the acceptance of that additional shortening. An inconspicuous lift in the shoe is often preferable to surgery, regardless of the low associated risks of surgical and anesthetic complications.

The same applies to angular deformities. Most angular deformities can be corrected manually. When this is not possible, internal fixation becomes the treatment of choice. In those instances when the angular deformity falls outside the recommended <10 degrees but is considered to be acceptable by the patient and surgeon, it is best to delay the introduction of weight bearing until intrinsic stability at the fracture site has taken place. Varus deformity is usually best tolerated by most people, particularly by men, because they usually have a built-in medial bowing of the tibia (Figs. 3.5 to 3.6). Women often have a mild valgus attitude of their knees. If this valgus is associated with a traumatic valgus angulation at the fracture site, the deformity may become evident. Under these circumstances, efforts should be made to reduce the angular deformity to a minimum.

There is ample documented evidence that 7 degrees of angulation at the fracture site is cosmetically acceptable and does not produce late osteoarthritic changes in the knee or ankle joints (11). Greater angulation may be cosmetically acceptable in some instances (Fig. 3.6). The compensatory motion provided by the subtalar joints helps alleviate the additional stresses placed at the tibiotalar joint. Even though the subtalar joint is capable of compensating best for valgus tibial angulation, we prefer the acceptance of a few degrees of varus rather than valgus. A varus deformity of a few degrees is often difficult to detect.

Angular deformity visible on the sagittal plane (antevarum and recurvatum), if only a few degrees, is functionally and cosmetically acceptable. As it is true with angular deformity in the coronal plane, most deformities are preventable and correctable by nonsurgical means. Recurvatum is easily produced during the application of the initial cast, particularly when the initial cast holds the ankle in plantar flexion (Figs. 3.8 and 3.9).

INDICATIONS AND CONTRAINDICATIONS

As indicated in the above section, closed diaphyseal tibial fractures experience, at the time of the injury, the final and total amount of shortening. In the case of axially unstable fractures, attempts to regain length by manipulation alone are likely to result in loss of the gained length upon the introduction of weight-bearing stresses. Even the active contraction of the ankle and toe flexors and extensors may produce the same result (37–38). This information suggests that axially unstable fracture of the tibial diaphysis that experiences unacceptable shortening at the time of the initial injury should not be treated with early bracing techniques. If activity can be postponed until intrinsic stability develops at the fracture site, then bracing can be carried out. Another option is the use of skeletal traction to the extremity until such stability is attained. External fixators can accomplish the same goal but should not be kept in place for too long a period of time. The rigid immobilization of the tibial fragments delays the healing of the tibia while allowing the fibular fracture to progress to healing in a rapid fashion. When the fixator is removed and weight bearing is introduced, the healed fibular fracture may lead to a varus deformity, as the tibia, still ununited, has failed to develop the necessary stability to prevent the deformity.

If a fracture that meets the criteria for functional bracing cannot be successfully aligned, surgical treatment should be instituted. Intramedullary nailing is a very effective method of treatment in many instances. Its use requires accurate knowledge of the technology involved in its performance and an awareness of its limitations. Recent literature has indicated that in many instances, particularly in fractures located in the proximal and distal thirds of the diaphysis, complications frequently occur by the creation and perpetuation of angular deformities, compartment syndromes may be created during the

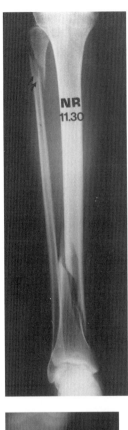
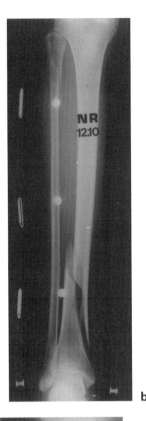

a

b

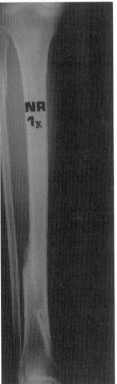
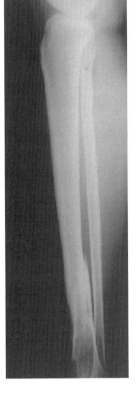

c, d

FIGURE 3.1. Composite photograph demonstrates the typical initial shortening seen in closed fractures of the tibia and fibula (**A**). The alignment seen after application of above-the-knee cast is shown. No attempt was made to regain the initially lost length (**B**). Radiograph was obtained 10 days after the initial insult, following the application of a functional brace (**C**). The fracture healed with abundant peripheral callus, in good alignment, and without additional shortening (**D**).

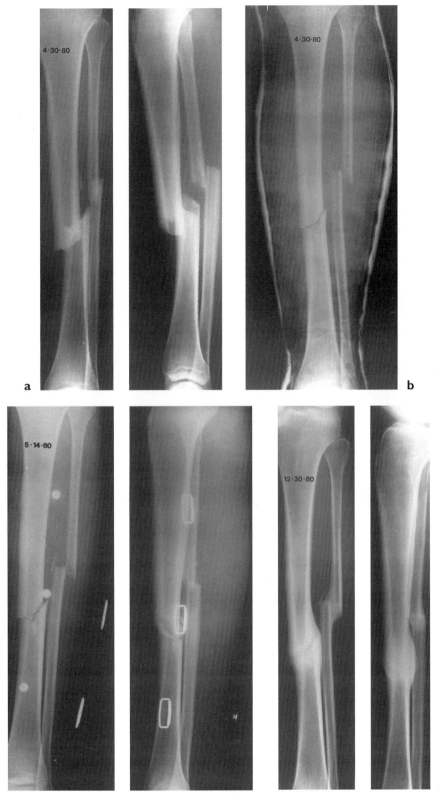

FIGURE 3.2. Minimally oblique fracture of the middle third of the tibia was associated with a fibular fracture (**A**). The fracture was manually reduced under anesthesia and stabilized in an above-the-knee cast (**B**). The cast was replaced with a below-the-knee functional brace 2 weeks later (**C**). The fracture healed uneventfully with good alignment of the fragments (**D**).

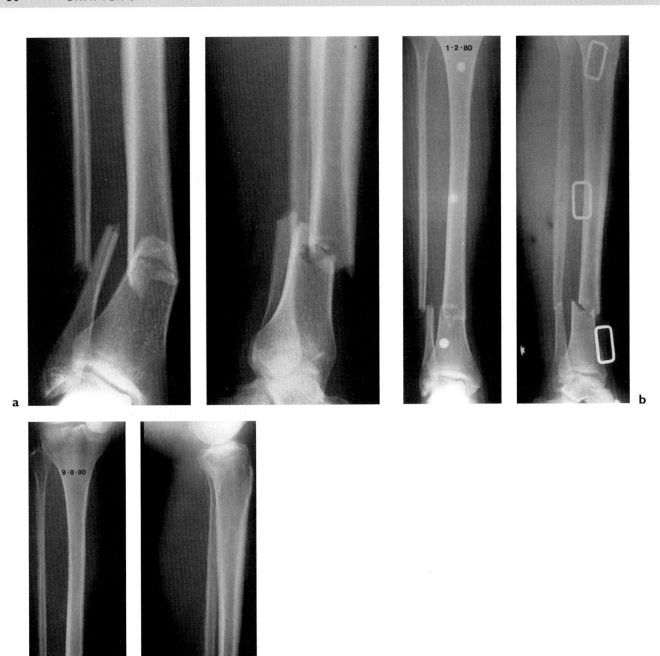

FIGURE 3.3. Transverse fractures of the tibia and fibula with significant angulation are shown (**A**). The fracture was reduced by manipulation under anesthesia (**B**). Two weeks later, the above-the-knee cast was replaced with a functional below-the-knee brace. The fracture healed uneventfully with a few degrees of anterior bowing (**C**).

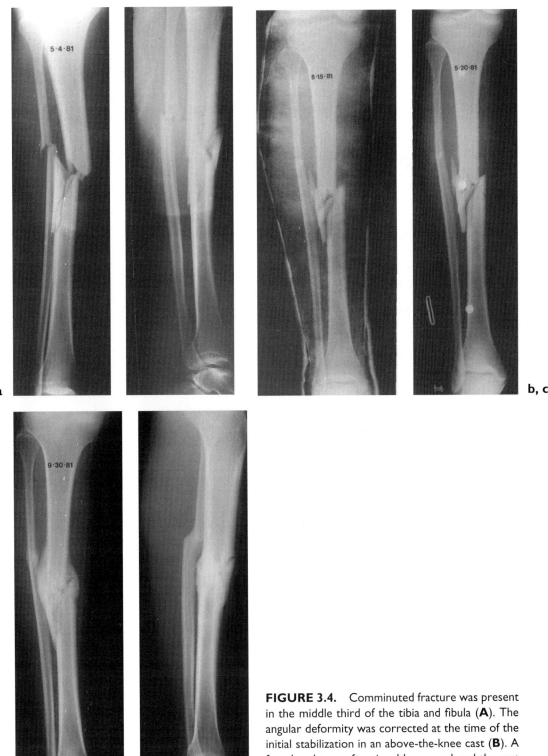

FIGURE 3.4. Comminuted fracture was present in the middle third of the tibia and fibula (**A**). The angular deformity was corrected at the time of the initial stabilization in an above-the-knee cast (**B**). A few days later, a functional brace replaced the cast (**C**). The fracture healed with a few degrees of varus angulation (**D**).

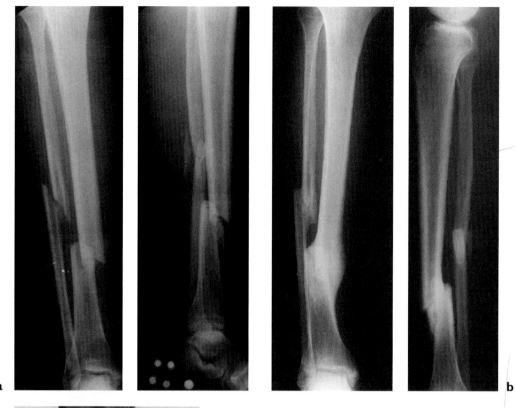

a   b

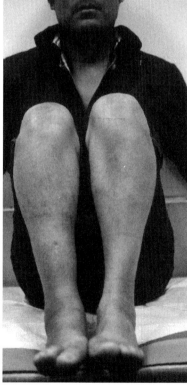

c

FIGURE 3.5. Transverse fracture of the tibia was incompletely reduced (**A**). A brace was applied, but the fracture healed with a moderately severe varus angulation (**B**). Clinical appearance of the varus angular deformity is presented (**C**). Incompletely reduced transverse fractures of the tibia are the ones most likely to develop varus deformity. With these fractures, if a stable reduction cannot be achieved, intramedullary fixation is the treatment of choice.

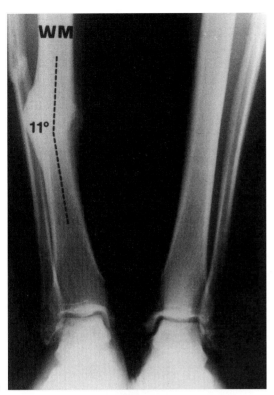

a

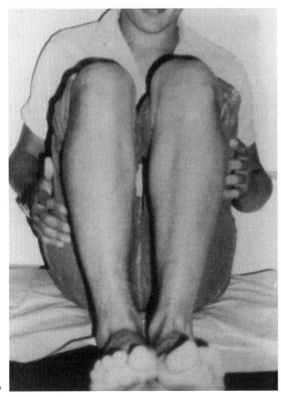

b

FIGURE 3.6. Fracture of the tibia and fibula healed with 11 degrees of varus (**A**). The history suggested that the patient had discontinued the brace when the symptoms disappeared and before consolidation of the fracture. From an aesthetic point of view, the deformity was acceptable (**B**).

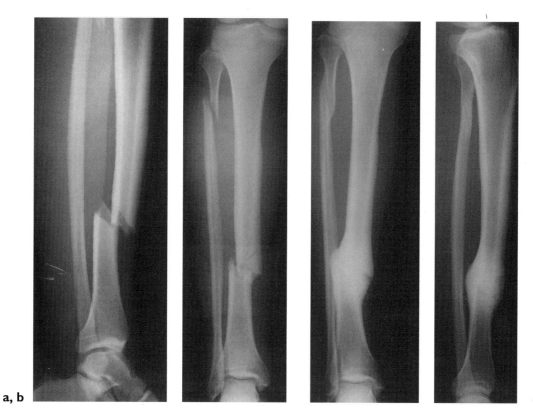

a, b   c

FIGURE 3.7. Transverse fracture of the tibia (**A**) was appropriately reduced and made stable (**B**). The fracture healed with a few degrees of angular deformity (**C**). Clinically, there was no cosmetic abnormality.

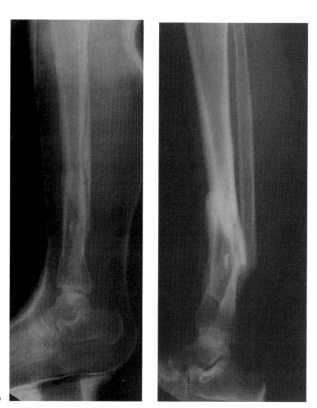

a, b

FIGURE 3.8. Fracture of the distal tibia and fibula was mistakenly stabilized in a cast with the ankle in plantar flexion (**A**). When the cast was replaced with a brace, weight was borne on the head of the metatarsals, forcing the fracture to angulate into recurvatum (**B**).

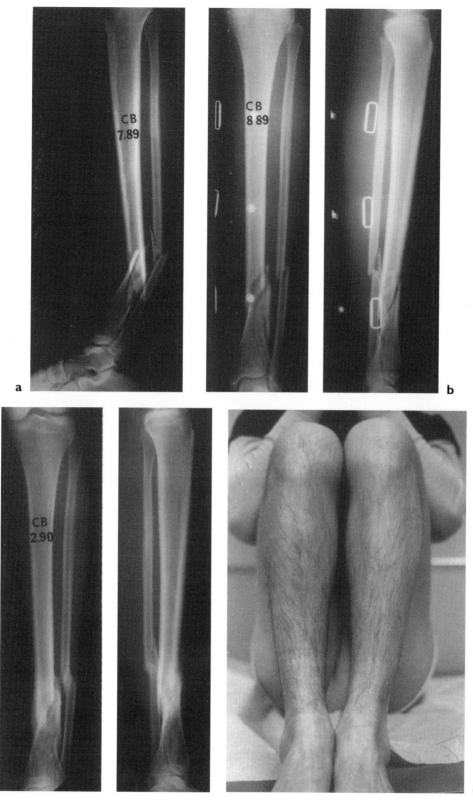

FIGURE 3.9. Comminuted fracture in the distal third of the tibia was associated with severe recurvatum (**A**). The angular deformity was corrected at the time of the initial stabilization in an above-the-knee cast. The cast was replaced with a functional brace within the next 2 weeks (**B**). The fracture healed without an angular deformity (**C**). The patient illustrates the overall appearance of his legs (**D**).

insertion of the nail, interlocking screws frequently break, and residual knee pain is a very common sequela. This latter problem often persists even after the removal of the intramedullary nail (11).

Transverse fractures that can be manipulated and rendered stable can be treated with functional braces, providing the reduction is a secure one (Fig. 3.3).

The presence of associated fibular fracture is almost always desirable. An intact fibula may produce a varus angular deformity upon the initiation of weight-bearing ambulation. In fractures located in the proximal or distal thirds of the tibial diaphysis, this complication is more likely to take place, particularly if the initial radiograph demonstrates angulation (Fig. 3.10).

If the fracture is located in the middle third of the tibial shaft and the initial radiograph shows a very mild varus angulation, a progression of the deformity is unlikely. With an intact fibula and an axially unstable fracture located in the proximal third, a deformity may occur. Closed tibial fractures located in the proximal third, which have an associated fibular fracture, can be, in most instances, successfully treated with functional braces (Figs. 3.11 and 3.12).

Fractures of the distal third of the tibia without an associated fibular fracture can also angulate into varus when weight bearing is introduced, particularly if they are oblique. These fractures, if initially angulated, are a definitive contraindication for functional bracing (Figs. 3.13 and 3.14). In general, the condition of the fibula should dictate whether a closed tibia fracture might be successfully treated by closed functional means.

Open fractures are usually accompanied by an initially greater degree of shortening. Therefore, functional bracing has a more limited role to play in their management. In general, only type I open fractures produced by lower energy forces can be considered appropriate subjects for functional bracing. Among them are fractures resulting from low-velocity gunshot wounds, when the initial shortening is acceptable. However, if shortening is to be accepted and its compensation with a shoe lift is a desirable option, bracing can be carried out, but usually after a longer period of stabilization in an above-the-knee cast. In the presence of significant swelling, it is best to delay the application of the weight-bearing cast or brace until the swelling has decreased significantly and the acute symptoms have also subsided. Failure to follow these criteria may result in an angular deformity. In special circumstances such as closed fractures associated with shortening considered to be outside the arbitrarily agreed-upon 12 mm, a few additional millimeters of shortening can be justified.

ACUTE MANAGEMENT

CLOSED FRACTURES

Closed diaphyseal tibial fractures resulting from low-energy forces do not, as a rule, require hospitalization. However, even if produced from rather mild trauma, hospitalization is recommended if the extremity is very swollen and painful after initial stabilization. Any signs or symptoms that suggest the possibility of a muscle compartment syndrome in the making require careful consideration. Hospitalization for an overnight observation is strongly recommended. Otherwise, a period of observation in an emergency room area is sufficient.

After appropriate sedation and upon confirmation of negative neurologic or vascular associated pathology, the injured extremity is stabilized in an above-the-knee cast that maintains the knee in no more than 7 degrees of flexion and the ankle in a neutral attitude of 90 degrees. The initial cast should be well padded to permit the unavoidable swelling that accompanies all fractures.

For patients with fractures associated with minimal soft tissue pathology, a strong narcotic is necessary before any attempts to stabilize the injured limb are made. Then, an above-the-knee cast is applied.

OPEN FRACTURES

All patients with open fractures must be admitted to the hospital. Not all of them need debridement in the operating room. Those produced by low-velocity bullet wounds that demonstrate a skin defect no greater than the small entry point of the projectile may be treated in the emergency room by appropriate cleansing of the wound and splinting. Nonetheless, at this time, it is best to admit these patients to the hospital for a 3-day observation time and administration of intravenous antibiotics. It is possible that some time in the near future, new oral antibiotics may be strong enough to make possible their administration through that route.

MANIPULATION

True manipulation is rarely necessary in the management of closed diaphyseal tibial fractures that are to be eventually treated with functional braces, except for those that are transverse and displaced. Axially unstable fractures (oblique, spiral, and comminuted) that demonstrate initial acceptable shortening do not need manipulation, but simply gentle alignment of the fragments. Satisfactory alignment can be obtained in most instances by simply allowing the injured extremity to hang freely over the side of the table on which the patient is either sitting or lying. At the time of application of the cast, further improvements in alignment can be obtained manually. The same applies to segmental fractures that demonstrate acceptable initial shortening and alignment. It is commonly accepted that segmental fractures are to be treated surgically. This is not necessarily true. If the initial shortening is acceptable, the middle fragment is not significantly displaced and can be manually aligned, and the knee and ankle joints can be made parallel to each other, the closed method of treatment may be instituted (Figs. 3.15 to 3.17; also see Fig. 3.24).

INITIAL IMMOBILIZATION

The initial means of immobilization is usually that provided by a well-padded above-the-knee cast, which, as indicated earlier, should hold the knee in no more than 7 degrees of flexion and the ankle at 90 degrees. It is mistakenly believed by some that the initial cast used to stabilize tibial fractures should hold the knee in a position of flexion to prevent shortening of the extremity. Obviously, this is wrong as the initial shortening of the fractured limb does not increase above and beyond that experienced at the time of the initial insult. Furthermore, ambulation in an above-the-knee cast is very difficult, particularly for the elderly patient.

If significant swelling and pain are present at the fracture site or the fracture was produced from a high-energy injury, it is best to stabilize the extremity on a padded splint that avoids the circumferential wrapping of plaster of Paris. Frequent monitoring of the muscle compartments of the leg is required and appropriate action taken if the pressures become dangerously elevated. Upon confirmation of acceptable pressures and in the absence of disproportional pain, the circular above-the-knee cast can be applied.

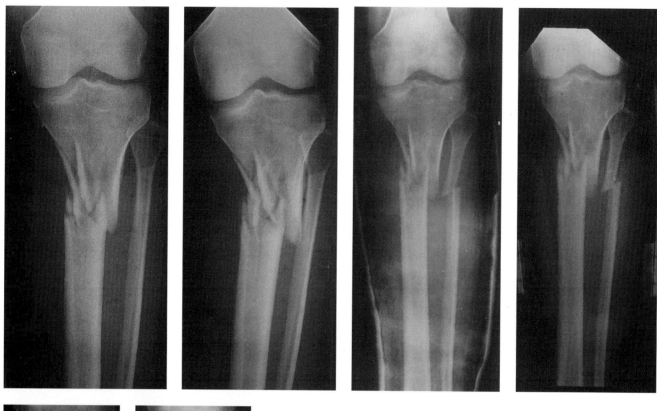

a, b

c, d

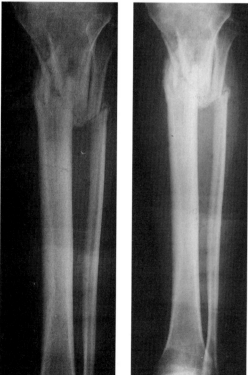

e, f

FIGURE 3.10. Comminuted fracture of the proximal tibia is shown. The absence of an associated fibular fracture was not recognized, and a functional brace was mistakenly applied (**A**). The fracture readily angulated into severe varus (**B**). An osteotomy of the fibula was performed, and the deformity was corrected. Radiographs demonstrate the correction of the deformity in the postoperative above-the-knee cast (**C**) and subsequently in a functional brace (**D**). Uneventful healing progressed (**E**). The fracture eventually healed with acceptable shortening and alignment (**F**).

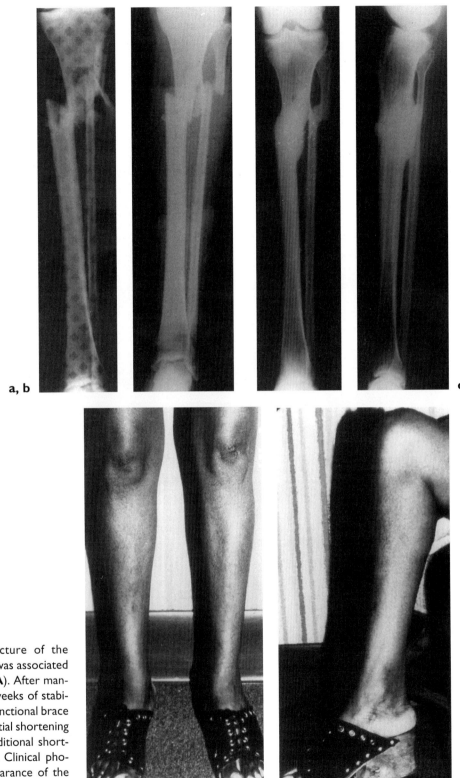

FIGURE 3.11. Comminuted fracture of the proximal third of the tibia and fibula was associated with marked translatory deformity (**A**). After manual reduction of the fracture and 3 weeks of stabilization in an above-the-knee cast, a functional brace was applied. Notice the acceptable initial shortening (**B**). The fracture healed without additional shortening and acceptable alignment (**C**). Clinical photographs depict the acceptable appearance of the injured extremity (**D and E**).

a, b

c

d, e

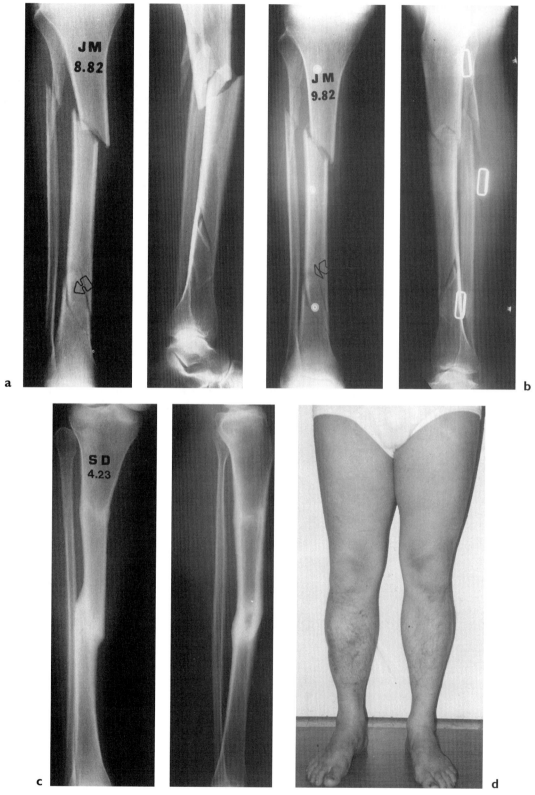

FIGURE 3.12. Segmental fracture of the tibia demonstrates a valgus deformity at the level of the proximal fracture (**A**). Approximately 3 weeks later, a functional brace was fitted (**B**). The fracture healed with an acceptable alignment of the fragments (**C**). The appearance of the lower extremities is presented (**D**).

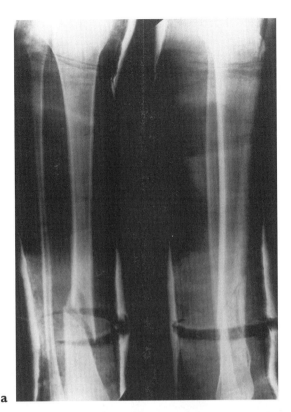

a

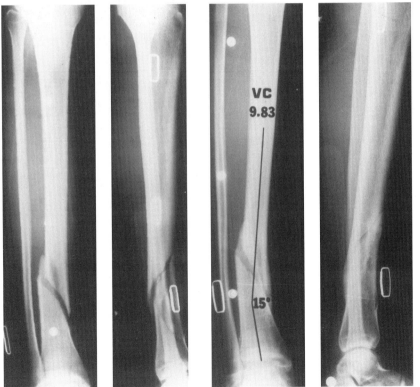

b   c

FIGURE 3.13.   Oblique fracture of the distal tibia was without an associated fracture of the fibula. Unrealistic attempts to correct the varus and rotary deformity were unsuccessful (**A**). A brace was mistakenly applied, and the deformity increased (**B**). The fracture healed with an obvious deformity (**C**). Oblique angulated fractures of the distal tibia, not associated with fibular fracture, should not be braced. The deformity is likely to increase with the introduction of weight-bearing stresses.

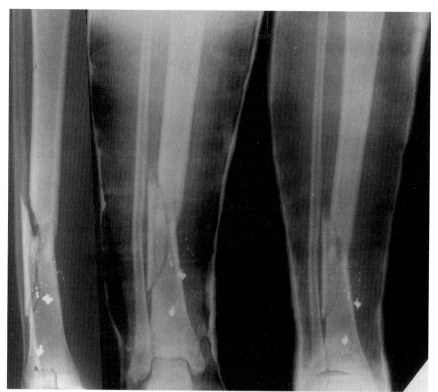

a, b, c

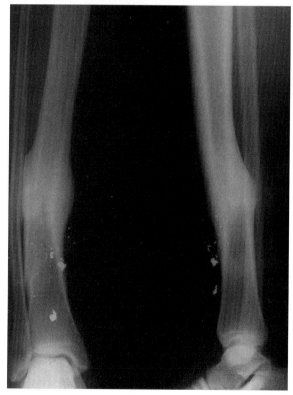

d

FIGURE 3.14. Comminuted fracture of the distal tibia without an associated fibular fracture is shown (**A**). Despite two attempts to correct the deformity, it persisted (**B and C**). The fracture healed in varus (**D**). These types of fractures should be managed with an ostectomy of the fibula or by means of internal fixation.

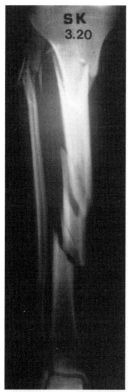

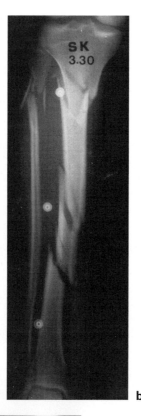

a

b

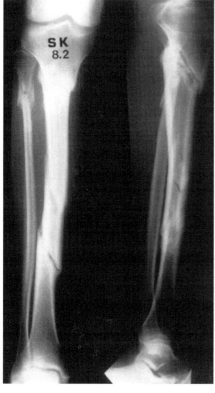

c

FIGURE 3.15. Double segmental fracture of the tibia and fibula was associated with minimal initial shortening or angulation (**A**). Ten days after the initial insult, a prefabricated functional brace was fitted (**B**). The fracture healed uneventfully, without additional shortening or angulation (**C**).

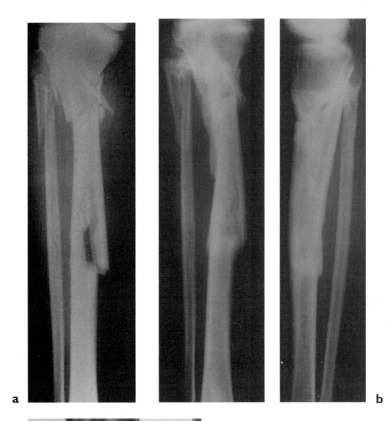

a   b

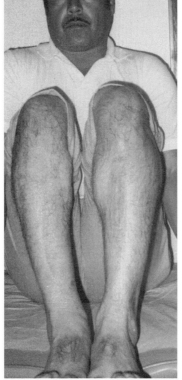

c

FIGURE 3.16. Segmental, comminuted fracture of the tibia and fibula was treated with a functional brace after initial stabilization in an above-the-knee cast (**A**). The fracture healed with acceptable length and alignment (**B**). The patient demonstrates the overall appearance of his lower extremities (**C**).

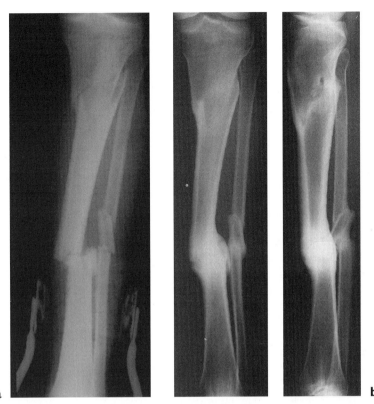

FIGURE 3.17. Segmental fracture of the tibia and fibula is presented. The fracture was treated with a custom-made functional brace (**A**). The fracture healed with acceptable length and alignment (**B**).

Manipulation of tibial fractures in the presence of significant swelling and pain should be avoided as it may precipitate the development of a compartment syndrome. After a fracture, particularly if it is displaced and shortened, the geometry of the extremity changes from that of a conical structure to one where the circumference of the limb at the fracture site increases. This change accommodates the increased fluid volume created by bleeding and bone marrow extravasation into the area. Sudden traction to the extremity forces increased pressures around the fracture, often sufficient to convert a benign situation into a full-blown compartment syndrome (34).

PATIENT INSTRUCTIONS

After the application of the above-the-knee cast, it is best to recommend a period of bed rest that ordinarily should not exceed 24 hours. During this period of time, the extremity should be held in an elevated position. The patient should be encouraged to carry out frequent isometric exercises to all muscle groups in the extremity, particularly the flexors and extensors of the ankle and toes. These exercises assist in preventing thromboembolic complications and produce motion at the fracture site, which has been proved to be beneficial to fracture repair (22,38,39). After the recommended period of relative rest in the above-the-knee cast, ambulation with aid of a walker or crutches should begin.

As, in closed fractures, shortening does not increase above and beyond that experienced at the time of the initial insult, there is no need to curtail the degree of weight bearing to which the patient can subject the fractured limb upon the initiation of ambulation. Symptoms should dictate the degree of activity. We feel, however, that patients who functionally use their injured extremities early regain comfortable ambulation sooner that those who, from fear of pain, delay function and weight-bearing ambulation.

It is likely that early ambulation reduces the severity of distal swelling. However, it is essential that the injured limb not be allowed to be dependent for long periods of time. We strongly recommend frequent short walks, followed by elevation of the extremity and continuation of isometric muscle exercises.

The above-the-knee cast is removed and replaced with a below-the-knee functional brace as soon as the acute symptoms and signs have subsided. This period of time varies from patient to patient and is influenced by the severity of the injury and individual personality and pain tolerance. The majority of patients who experience low-energy injuries find it possible to receive the brace before the end of the second week after injury. However, if at that time there are still significant distal swelling and pain at the fracture site, an additional week of ambulation in the above-the-knee cast is recommended.

FOLLOW-UP

After application of the functional brace and radiologic confirmation of an acceptable relationship between the fracture fragments, the patient is instructed on the appropriate tightening of the Velcro straps to ensure that the brace fits snugly at all times. The inevitable reduction of edema and increased muscle atrophy result in a loss of the tight fit of the brace, necessary for the maintenance of alignment of the fragments. The brace then has a tendency to slip distally. Therefore, patients should adjust the straps on a regular basis. The frequency of this maneuver decreases as the tissues stabilize themselves. During recumbency, patients may remove their shoes; however, the dorsal Velcro strap must be adjusted to prevent distal slippage of the brace.

Instructions regarding temporary removal of the brace are not given to patients until 1 week has elapsed and new radiographs are obtained. This is a precautionary measure we have long practiced in order to prevent as much as possible improper premature donning and doffing of the brace.

EXPECTED OUTCOME

The vast majority of closed diaphyseal tibial fractures are expected to heal uneventfully. Our nonunion rate in a group of 1,000 fractures was 1.5%. As the initial shortening of closed tibial fractures is around 1 cm in most instances, the final shortening in that particular group was <12 mm in 95% of the patients (39). It is likely that if we had been more aware of the behavior of tibial fractures from the beginning of the series, we would have been more careful in the selection of patients for functional bracing.

If the alignment of the fracture is acceptable after the application of the brace and angular deformity does not exceed 5 degrees, the final angulation should be expected to be within a functionally and cosmetically acceptable range. In the series of patients mentioned above, 95% of the patients had healing of their fractures with <8 degrees of angulation. Ninety-two percent had <6 degrees of angulation.

These criteria also apply to segmental fractures. If the initial shortening was acceptable and the obtained alignment of the fragments satisfactory, functional bracing is likely to be successful (see Figs. 3.15 to 3.17).

Open fractures, the result of low-energy injury, which demonstrate minimal initial shortening and moderate soft tissue pathology, may be braced, but the period of stabilization in an above-the-knee cast or an external fixator must be longer than that desirable for closed low-energy fractures. In the case of open fractures, oftentimes it is necessary to accept a degree of shortening slightly greater than in closed fractures (Figs. 3.18 to 3.20). It must be kept in mind that a great deal of progress has been made in the area of closed intramedullary fixation of long bone fractures. The open fracture is the fracture that has benefited most from this improved technology.

Patient cooperation is necessary to obtain the best possible clinical results. Premature removal of the brace or failure to maintain the snug fit of the brace, particularly during the first few weeks, may allow angular deformities to develop.

If the brace is applied during the first few weeks after the initial insult, one can expect no limitation of motion of any of the joints in the injured extremity. The time of stabilization in the above-the-knee cast, being as short as we have indicated, is not sufficient to create permanent limitation of motion. We have confirmed that whatever limitation of joint motion is measured at the time of removal of the brace spontaneously disappears within a short period of time.

Though a percentage of patients have a permanent degree of angular deformity or shortening of the injured extremity, late degenerative joint disease is not likely to develop. The literature is rich in well-documented studies demonstrating that the body is capable of tolerating angular tibial deformities with impunity. We have personally never seen a patient develop arthritis of the knee or ankle after a tibial diaphyseal fracture that healed with angulation.

Rotary deformities may be found in healed tibial fractures. Experiences have shown us that such deformities are usually the result of failure to correct the deformity that develops immediately after the fracture occurs, during the application of the initial cast. If no rotary deformity is present at the time of application of the brace and the brace is appropriately worn, a rotary deformity is not likely to occur. We demonstrated in clinical experimental studies that the malrotation at the fracture site that occurs early during weight-bearing ambulation spontaneously corrects itself during the swing phase of gait (38). A rotary deformity of <10 degrees is rarely noticed during ambulation (Fig. 3.21).

MANAGING COMPLICATIONS

LATE NERVE PALSY

Injury to the peroneal nerve is not uncommon in diaphyseal tibial fractures, particularly when a proximal fibula fracture also occurs. In most instances, the deep peroneal branch of the sciatic nerve is injured. Spontaneous recovery cannot be taken for granted. If recovery is to occur, it usually requires a very long period of time. Electrical testing may be carried out. Magnetic resonance imaging studies can, in most instances, confirm the type of nerve injury, permitting in that manner an appropriate therapeutic protocol.

Injury to the posterior tibial nerve is rare in association with closed diaphyseal tibial fractures. Therefore, it is not likely to be seen in patients managed with functional braces.

Late peroneal palsy may be the result of excessive pressure exerted by the superior brim of the brace against the neck of the fibula. This complication is preventable by careful fit of the brace and inspection of the area during the early days after the application of the orthotic device. Trimming of the extended

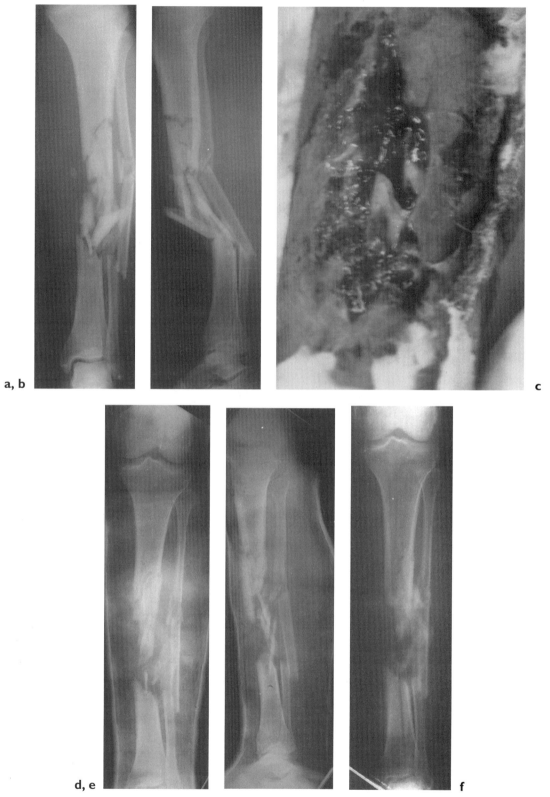

a, b

c

d, e

f

FIGURE 3.18.   Open comminuted fracture of the tibia was the result of a severe crushing injury (**A and B**). Upon admission to our hospital 1 week later, the wound was debrided and a large bony fragment removed (**C**). Subsequently, a functional below-the-knee cast was applied (**D and E**). Two weeks later, the cast was removed and a custom-made below-the-knee brace was applied (**F**). *Continued.*

FIGURE 3.18. *Continued* The fracture healed with acceptable alignment and length (**G**). The patient demonstrates the appearance of the injured extremity. The wound healed without the need for skin surgery (**H**).

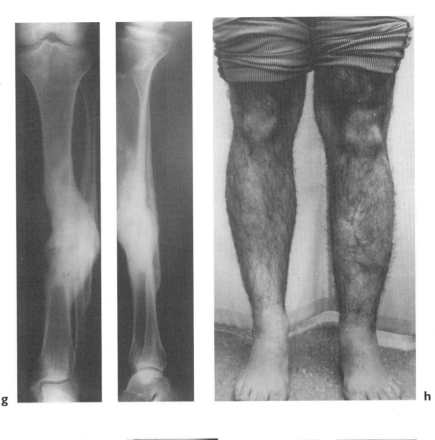

g

h

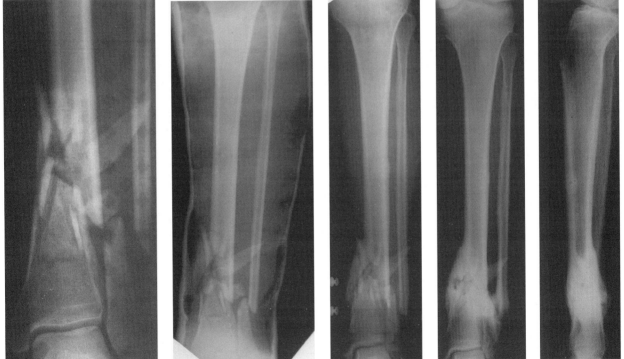

a, b, c

d

FIGURE 3.19. Open comminuted fracture of the distal tibia and fibula (**A**) was treated by debridement and stabilization in a weight-bearing above-the-knee cast (**B**). A few weeks later, the cast was replaced with a brace (**C**). The fracture healed with acceptable shortening and angulation (**D**).

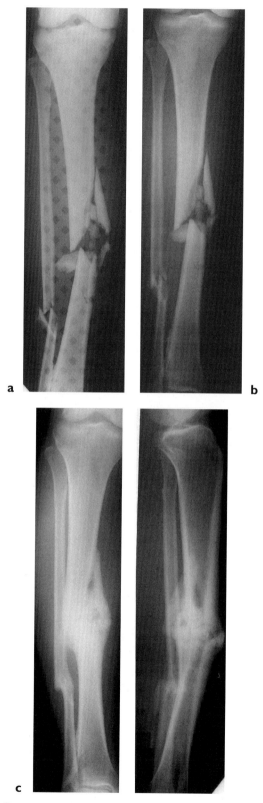

FIGURE 3.20.   Open comminuted fracture of the tibia and fibula was the result of a high-energy injury (**A**). Though fractures of this type are not frequently managed with early functional bracing, a brace was erroneously applied in this instance (**B**). The fracture healed with shortening and angular deformities (**C**).

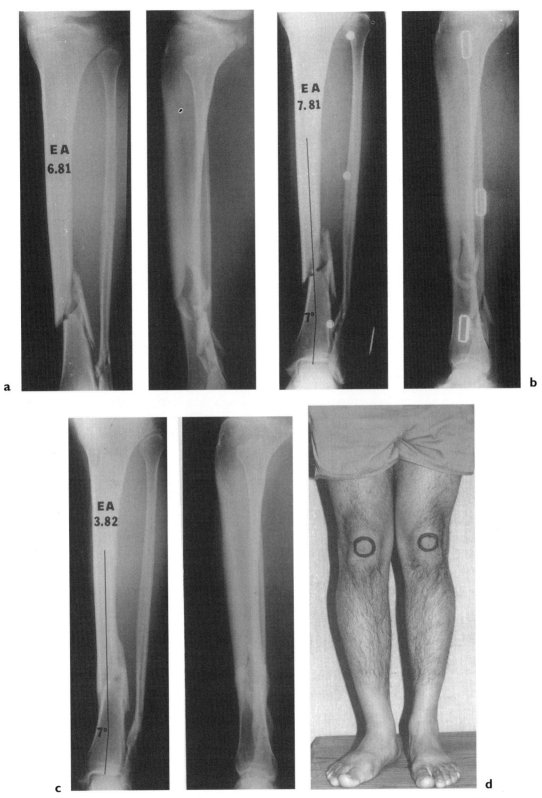

FIGURE 3.21.   Closed comminuted fracture of the distal tibia and fibula is shown (**A**). Notice the rotary deformity, as depicted by the wide space between the tibia and fibula. One month later, a brace was applied (**B**). The malrotation was not recognized, and therefore efforts to correct it were not made. The fracture healed with a few degrees of varus and a permanent external rotation deformity (**C**). The patient demonstrates the external rotation deformity, which he spontaneously compensates for when walking (**D**).

wing of the brace and relief of the compressed area should suffice. Spontaneous recovery should take place if the pressure was not sustained for a long period of time and was not of a severe degree.

MALALIGNMENT AND SHORTENING

The recognition of unacceptable alignment of the fracture fragments after the application of the initial cast is not always a mandate to abandon the closed treatment. A new cast can always be applied, and under anesthesia if necessary. If this second reduction does not render the desirable response, another treatment modality is usually necessary. Minor angular deformities are usually correctable either with cast wedging or during the application of a new cast, after the acute swelling subsides (Figs. 3.22 and 3.23).

A few degrees of initial malalignment is acceptable, provided it does not exceed 5 to 8 degrees. This angular deformity is usually easily corrected at the time of brace application. If such correction is not possible through this mechanism, recasting or surgical treatment becomes desirable or necessary. Individual discretion is necessary on the part of the treating physician.

There are times when shortening or angulation of greater degree is acceptable. One should not consider a failure of treatment the presence of a tibial fracture that occurs in a sedentary elderly individual that heals with 2 cm of shortening or 10 degrees of angulation. This shortening can be easily managed by the addition of a 1-cm lift to the shoe. The angular deformity is not likely to be noticeable and will not result in degenerative arthritis at a later date (11). The same rationale may be used in the care of virtually all patients if the infrastructure of the health services in a given area precludes the safe use of sophisticated surgical technology. One should keep in mind that before the modern era, fractures were treated by simple nonsurgical means and often with good functional results. Deviations from the normal, such as minor angular deformities and extremity shortening, did not prevent patients from returning to farming or other strenuous activities. It was not until aseptic surgical techniques, anesthesia, antibiotics, and improved metallurgy and imaging technology became available that the surgical fixation of fractures became a viable option.

As indicated before, intramedullary nailing is a very appropriate means of stabilization for open tibial fractures. The results thus far obtained have been very good in many instances, and frequently this treatment modality is the preferred one. As it is true for all known methods of treatment, intramedullary nailing is not a panacea. A number of complications have been acknowledged, among which pain over the proximal tibia is the one most troublesome. Some surgeons have reported the need for nail removal in a very high percentage of patients and a persistence of pain after nail removal in as many as 40% of the patients. Failure of the interlocking screws is also a frequent complication, for which difficult surgery is often necessary (Figs. 3.24 and 3.25) (11).

The presence of an intraarticular component of a distal tibial fracture does not necessarily call for a surgical intervention. Minimally displaced intraarticular fractures do well after early motion of the tibiotalar joint, followed by the introduction of gradually progressive weight-bearing ambulation (Figs. 3.26 to 3.28). Mild traumatic intraarticular incongruity is well tolerated by the joint, and the introduction of early function ensures preservation of normal articular cartilage (16–18).

DELAYED UNION AND NONUNION

See Chapter 4, Delayed Union and Nonunion, for details.

INITIAL STABILIZATION

The initial cast used to stabilize the fracture should extend from the base of the toes to midthigh. The knee is held in no more than 7 degrees of flexion and the ankle in a neutral attitude. Plantar flexion of the ankle must be carefully avoided. The extension of the knee makes early weight-bearing ambulation possible. An equinus deformity of the ankle can easily produce a recurvatum deformity of the fractured tibia when the cast is replaced with a brace that permits motion of all joints and graduated weight-bearing ambulation.

The initial above-the-knee cast must be padded to allow for additional swelling to take place.

After confirming the absence of warning signs of an impending compartment syndrome, the patient should be shown the appropriate use of crutches or walkers. Curtailment from weight bearing is not necessary because the initial shortening will not increase, as indicated earlier. Ambulation with crutches or a walker is recommended simply to prevent pain. Once the acute pain subsides, it is desirable to use the extremity as much as possible within the limits imposed by the degree of pain. Frequent periods of leg elevation and active use of the toes are recommended. They assist in the prevention of excessive swelling and expedite the disappearance of pain.

BELOW-THE-KNEE FUNCTIONAL CAST

After a period of time in the above-the-knee cast, a below-the-knee functional cast is applied. The time in the long leg cast is determined by the severity of the injury and associated physical findings. Fractures minimally displaced and the result of a low-energy injury may be transferred to the below-the-knee cast or brace within the first 2 weeks. Those patients who by that time are still experiencing significant pain and demonstrate distal swelling should be held in the above-the-knee cast for an additional 1 or 2 weeks. During this time, they should be encouraged to elevate the leg frequently, to do isometric exercises with the musculature of the leg, and to bear partial weight on the leg. These measures expedite recovery.

In the event that the surgeon wishes to use the below-the-knee functional cast in preference to the functional brace, the following steps must be followed. It is best to apply the first portion of the cast while the knee is flexed and hangs over the side of the table. The opposite extremity should be fully exposed to appreciate the overall alignment of the normal leg and therefore make possible the replication of its shape and contour on the fractured limb. This practice is most helpful for the prevention of rotary deformities. An assistant should hold the ankle at 90 degrees of dorsiflexion. While the ankle is held in that position, plaster is rolled over the foot and ankle joint (Figs. 3.29 and 3.30).

It is of the utmost importance not to stabilize the ankle in an equinus position. The ankle joint of a traumatized extremity becomes stiff within a short period of time. When the stabilizing cast is eventually removed, to be replaced with a brace that permits free motion of the ankle, the stiff joint forces the patient to bear weight, not within the normal sequence of heel strike, foot flat, and toe off phases but with an initial contact of the metatarsal heads with the ground. This contact results in a direct transfer of weight-bearing forces to the still-mobile fracture site, resulting in a recurvatum deformity (Fig. 3.8).

It is commonly believed that a recurvatum deformity is likely to occur in fractures of the distal third of the tibia. Though this is true to some extent, this complication is preventable in most instances. The deformity usually appears

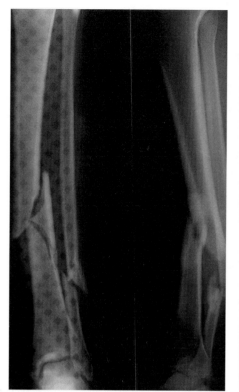

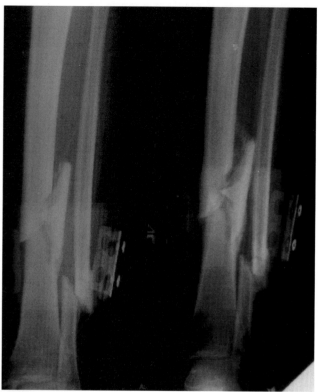

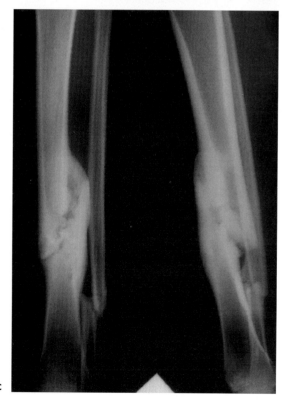

FIGURE 3.22. Closed comminuted fracture of the tibia and fibula is shown (**A**). The initial angular valgus and recurvatum deformities were corrected, and the limb was stabilized in an above-the-knee cast. Within 2 weeks, the cast was removed and replaced with a below-the-knee functional brace (**B**). The fracture healed without shortening above that present at the time of the injury (**C**).

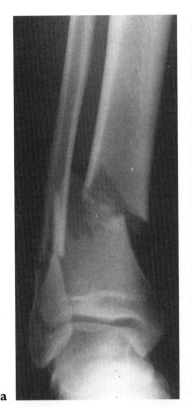
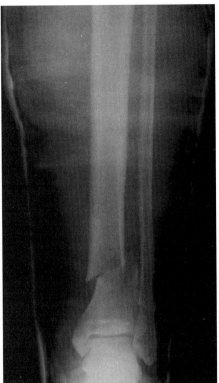
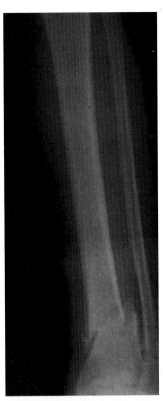

a

b, c

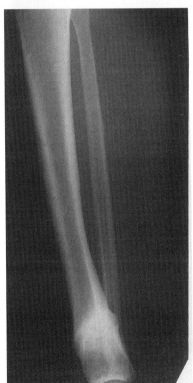
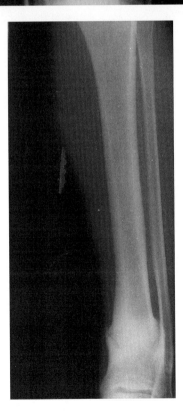

d

FIGURE 3.23. Slightly oblique fracture of the distal tibia and fibula (**A**) was initially stabilized in an above-the-knee cast. After manual correction of the deformity (**B**), a brace was applied. However, the fragments angulated into varus (**C**). The fractures healed with only minimal angular deformity (**D**).

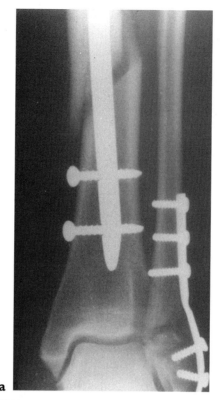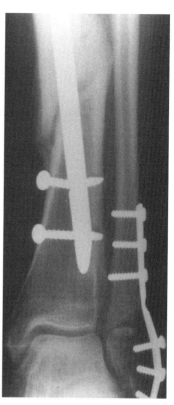

a   b

FIGURE 3.24.   Oblique fracture of the distal tibia and fibula was treated with inter-locking intramedullary nailing (**A**). The fracture healed after the interlocking screws broke and the fracture angulated into varus (**B**).

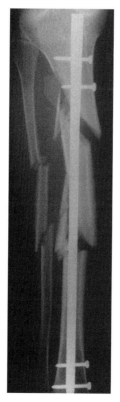

FIGURE 3.25.   Segmental fracture of the tibia was associated with a fibular fracture, which was treated with interlocking nail fixation. Though a widely accepted method of treatment, frac-tures of the proximal third are often difficult to nail without a resulting angular deformity.

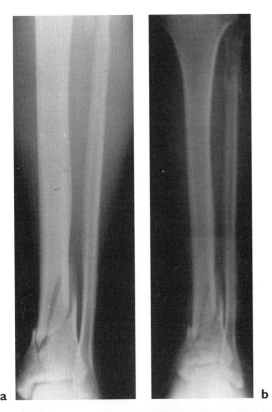

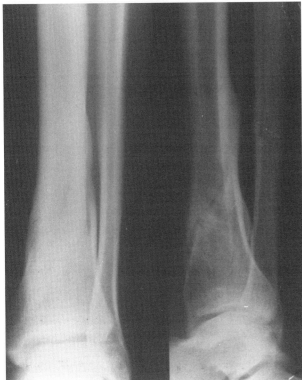

FIGURE 3.26. Slightly comminuted fracture of the distal tibia and proximal fibula with a likely intraarticular component (**A**) was treated with a functional brace after a couple of weeks of stabilization in an above-the-knee cast. The fracture showed acceptable alignment in the brace (**B**). The fracture healed uneventfully (**C**).

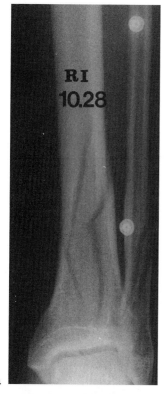
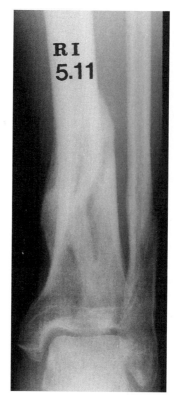
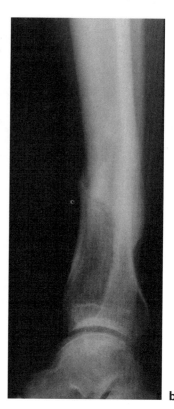

a

b

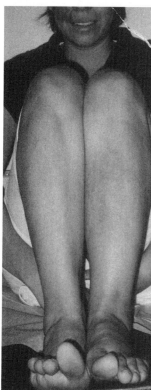

c

FIGURE 3.27.   Minimally displaced fracture of the distal end of the tibia and fibula is shown. The fracture probably extended into the joint (**A**). The fracture was treated in a functional below-the-knee brace and healed uneventfully (**B**). The clinical appearance of the lower extremities is also presented (**C**).

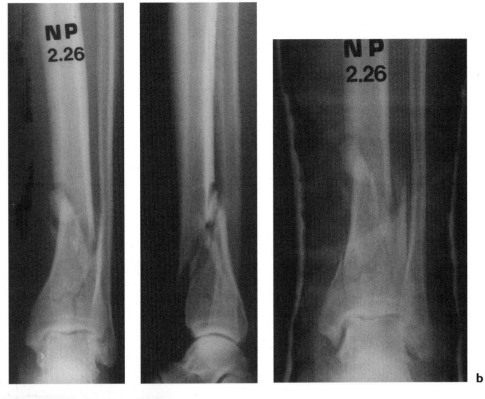

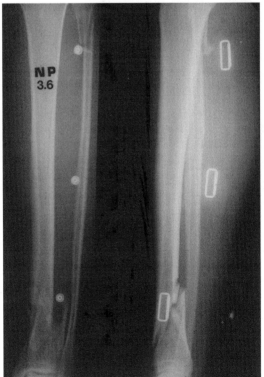

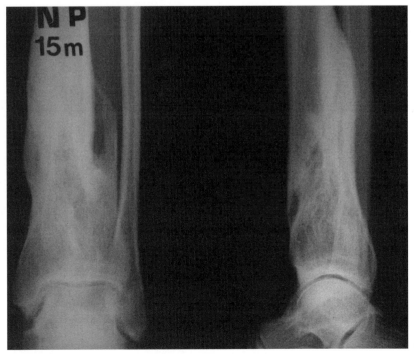

FIGURE 3.28. Mildly comminuted fracture of the distal tibia and proximal fibula was associated with an intraarticular component (**A**). After 2 weeks of stabilization in an above-the-knee cast (**B**), a below-the-knee prefabricated functional brace was applied (**C**). The fracture healed without displacement of the fragments and with full range of motion of the ankle joint (**D**).

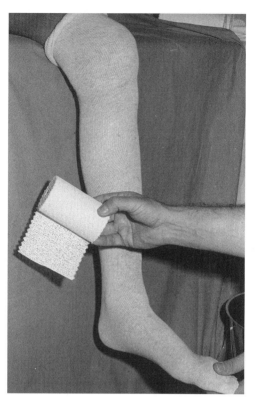

FIGURE 3.29. In the event the surgeon does not wish to use a brace that permits motion of the knee and ankle joints, a below-the-knee functional cast may be applied. The steps taken for the appropriate application of this cast require that the patient's legs rest freely over the side of a table with the hips, knees, and ankles at 90 degrees. Both legs must be exposed to ensure appropriate correction of angular and rotary deformities. This cast should follow the use of the initial well-padded above-the-knee cast that holds the knee in a few degrees of flexion and the ankle at 90 degrees. The skin is covered with a thin layer of stockinet. Padding with cotton wadding is optional. Before the wrapping of the stabilizing material, any rotary deformities must be corrected. Plaster of Paris or soft cast is wrapped over the foot and ankle, avoiding undue pressure over bony prominences.

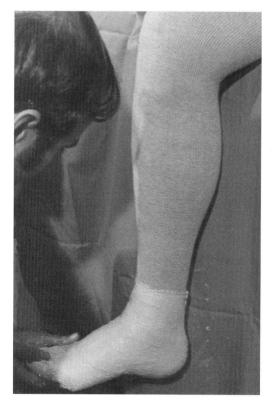

FIGURE 3.30. Notice that the ankle is gently held at 90 degrees of dorsiflexion.

when the initial cast is applied if the knee is held in extension. If the patient's knee and hip joints are held at 90 degrees of flexion and the patient has been anesthetized or heavily sedated, the common plantar flexion of the ankle can be gingerly corrected. This is why we think it is important to apply the cast in stages, where the ankle is addressed first and then the more proximal segments of the limb are stabilized (Fig. 3.9).

Once the ankle portion of the cast has begun to set, the cast is extended to the level of the tibial tubercle. It is during this time that the surgeon must obtain the best possible alignment of the fragments (Fig. 3.31). In axially unstable fractures, that is, oblique, spiral, and comminuted, no manipulation is necessary if the initial shortening is acceptable. However, if the fracture is axially unstable and the initial shortening is either unacceptable or borderline, but it appears that an anatomical reduction can be easily achieved by manipulation, such a reduction may be carried out. This reduction is traumatic and should be carried out under anesthesia at the time of the patient's initial visit to the emergency room. If a reduction cannot be achieved, then other approaches should be sought, such as stabilization with an external fixator or intramedullary fixation.

Once this second section of the cast has been completed, the knee should be extended to −45 degrees and the patient's heel allowed to rest on the surgeon's lap. The quadriceps must be relaxed (Fig. 3.32).

Plaster is then wrapped over the knee, extending just above the proximal pole of the patella (Fig. 3.33). As the plaster begins to harden, the surgeon applies moderate pressure over the relaxed patellar tendon (Figs. 3.33 to 3.35). Simultaneously, firm pressure is applied over the subpopliteal space. The condyles of the tibia and femur are also firmly molded.

As soon as the plaster appears to be moderately hard, it is trimmed to make possible full flexion and extension of the knee. The superior trimming should be at the level of the proximal pole of the patella and should extend in a transverse fashion to the hamstring tendons and posteriorly at a point approximately 1 in below the patellar tendon indentation (Fig. 3.36). Upon completion of the trimming procedure, the surgeon must ascertain that full flexion and extension of the knee will be possible (Fig. 3.37). The fact that the knee was held in 45 degrees of flexion during the wrapping of plaster over the knee joint ensures full extension of the knee. If plaster were wrapped while the knee was in 90 degrees of flexion, the patient would not be able to extend the joint because the proximal portion of the cast would cut into the patella.

Any pressure over the hamstring tendons must be eliminated.

A rubber heel can then be attached to the cast, being careful to avoid its positioning in ways that produce undue varus or valgus stresses on the knee joint. Once the plaster is completely dried, approximately 24 hours after its application, partial weight-bearing ambulation may be initiated (Fig. 3.38). The degree of weight borne on the extremity should be dictated by symptoms. Under no circumstances should patients be told to bear weight that produces pain. Initially, all patients experience discomfort upon beginning weight bearing. This discomfort decreases as activities become progressively greater. Eventually the pain disappears, making it possible for the patient to bear full weight.

New casting and bracing techniques have been recently developed in Europe and in the United States that have expanded the indications for the nonsurgical management of many fractures. These methods provide adequate stabilization to fractures while allowing greater stresses to be transferred to the fracture site. One of these developments is soft plaster.

The same protocol used for the application of the below-the-knee functional cast applies to all other modalities. Therefore, the indications and contraindication to bracing, timing of brace application, and postbracing management are the same.

APPLICATION OF FUNCTIONAL BRACE

The brace can be made of either plaster of Paris of the hard or soft type or of plastic materials. The plastic braces may be custom-made or prefabricated. In any event, it is important to recognize that the brace must be made adjustable in order to maintain the desirable snugness of the appliance. The adjustability of the brace makes it possible to compress the soft tissues at all times and in that manner perpetuates the hydraulic environment that controls angulation.

CUSTOM-MADE BRACE

If the brace is made of casting material, the technique used is identical to one described above for dealing with the below-the-knee functional cast. It is only the first stage (foot and ankle) of the casting that is eliminated. After a sock is applied over the patient's foot, a plastic insert is placed over the patient's heel and fastened to the cast with additional casting material. To make possible firm contact between the patient's leg and the brace, it is most desirable to split the cast posteriorly and remove a sliver of plaster approximately 1 in wide. This allows for adjustments to accommodate changes in the girth of the extremity (Fig. 3.39).

THERMOPLASTIC CUSTOM-MADE BRACE

Contrary to the technique of brace construction with wrapping materials, the Orthoplast (Johnson and Johnson) method calls for the use of a thermoplastic material. The Orthoplast sheet is a thin sheet of a synthetic rubber that, when dipped in hot water, softens for a few minutes before it once again reaches the preheated hard state.

The following steps are followed for the appropriate application of the custom-made below-the-knee functional Orthoplast brace. The patient must sit on a high table with the hips, knees, and ankles held at 90 degrees. Holding the knee in extension can create a posterior angular deformity.

The girth of the leg is measured at approximately the level of the apex of the gastrosoleus muscle and distally a couple of inches above the malleoli (Figs. 3.40 and 3.41). The length of the leg is measured from the proximal pole of the patella to 1 in below the lateral malleolus. These measurements are placed in front of the precut sheets of Orthoplast. The appropriate size of Orthoplast is then selected.

The selected sheet of Orthoplast is tentatively placed over the leg for a rough estimation of its eventual fit (Fig. 3.42). The plastic sheet is then dipped in hot water and held there for approximately 5 minutes. The heat softens the material and makes it pliable (Fig. 3.43). The leg has been previously covered with a single layer of stockinet.

Orthoplast material is placed directly over the extremity. The proximal end should be slightly over the proximal pole of the patella (Fig. 3.44). Then the material is wrapped over the leg, allowing its soft surfaces to overlap (Fig. 3.45). Premature contact between the surfaces of the material must be carefully avoided to prevent them from sticking together.

Gradual contact between the two surfaces is achieved carefully. Redundant "dog ears" are removed with the aid of scissors (Fig. 3.46).

Up to this point, the material is still soft and malleable. An elastic bandage saturated in cold water is firmly wrapped over the leg (Fig. 3.47). Then the surgeon carries out the necessary corrections in the axial and rotary alignment of the bones, carefully referring to the appearance of the exposed normal limb.

Within a few minutes, the Orthoplast material begins to harden. Before this happens, the surgeon molds the medial condylar surface and the antero-medial aspect of the tibial shaft. The patellar tendon is also compressed to resemble the patellar tendon indentation of the patella tendon bearing (PTB) prosthesis worn by the below-the-knee amputee (Fig. 3.48). Excessive material proximally and distally can be trimmed with scissors until full range of motion of the knee and ankle is possible (Fig. 3.49).

The foot plastic insert is then placed over the patient's heel, and the proximal uprights are brought in contact with the Orthoplast sleeve (Fig. 3.50). They are held in place with a strip of softened Orthoplast. To further reinforce the bond between the approximated surfaces of the plastic materials, their surfaces should be moistened with carbon tetrachloride before coming in contact with each other (Fig. 3.51).

The flexible uprights of the foot insert permit the donning and doffing of socks (Fig. 3.52). The dorsal Velcro strap over the dorsum of the foot prevents the slippage of the "sleeve" during the night, when the shoe is not in place (Fig. 3.52).

The Orthoplast brace can be made removable, facilitating in that manner the desirable adjustments prompted by the reduction of swelling that occurs after the introduction of function. To make the brace removable, the plastic sleeve is split posteriorly using a cast saw. A 0.5-in strip of material is removed, and Velcro straps are attached to the surface of the brace (Fig. 3.53).

PREFABRICATED BRACE

There are a number of prefabricated tibial braces on the market. What is most important in choosing a brace is an understanding of the philosophy and rationale of the method and the implementation of the treatment.

The following illustrations depict the steps to be taken in selecting the appropriate brace size and its application. It is essential that both lower extremities be exposed in order for the surgeon to attempt the reproduction of the shape and alignment of the noninjured extremity in the injured leg (Fig. 3.54). Though this preparatory step should have been taken at the time of the original stabilization of the fracture, there are times when the treating physician does not know if such a step was appropriately taken by the original physician.

On rare occasions, a patient demonstrates in the nonfractured leg angular or rotary deformities that preclude the use of a prefabricated brace. Radiologic views in combination with visual observation of the two limbs make it possible, in most instances, to determine whether or not the alignment of the fractured limb is acceptable.

A feature that is often inappropriately ignored is that of rotation of the fragments. As is true for the other important parameters, correction of rotary deformities is best obtained at the time of the initial stabilization in the above-the-knee cast. Most tibial fractures with an associated fibular fracture experience an external rotation deformity. Those with an intact fibula are more likely to experience an internal rotation. It is obvious that if the rotary deformities are not corrected before application of the brace, the deformity will become a permanent one.

That was the case illustrated in Fig. 3.21. Notice that an external rotation deformity was present in the initially stabilizing above-the-knee cast. The

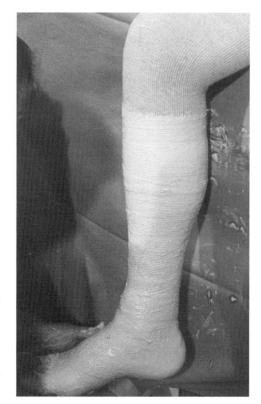

FIGURE 3.31. Once the plaster begins to set over the foot and ankle, the leg is wrapped with the same material. The plaster should be firmly wrapped over the soft tissues of the leg. It is at this time that any angular deformities may be corrected.

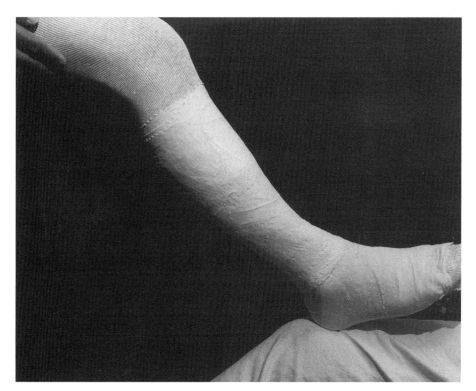

FIGURE 3.32. Once the second stage of plaster has hardened, the knee is extended to approximately 45 degrees of flexion. The patient's heel should rest on the surgeon's lap.

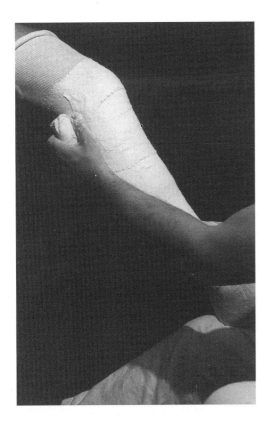

FIGURE 3.33. Plaster is then wrapped over the proximal tibia, extending to just above the femoral condyles.

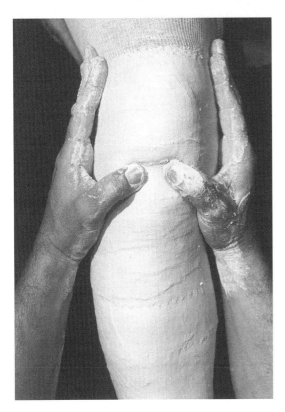

FIGURE 3.34. The medial tibial condyle and popliteal areas are very firmly compressed. As soon as the plaster begins to harden, the surgeon firmly molds the femoral condyles and patellar tendon.

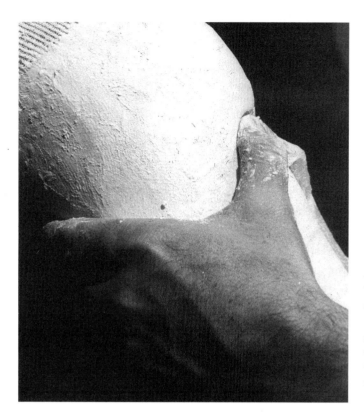

FIGURE 3.35. The patient must relax the quadriceps to make possible the indentation over the patellar tendon. The indentation does not require very strong pressure that could create damage to the underlying skin. The patellar tendon is not a major weight-bearing area; it simply assists in narrowing the upper mouth of the cast to provide angular and lateral stability to the fracture. The high "wings" assist in providing angular and rotary stability to the fracture.

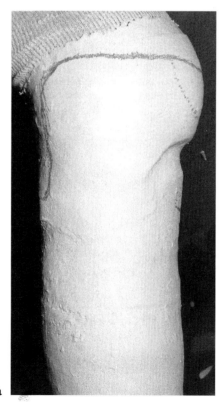

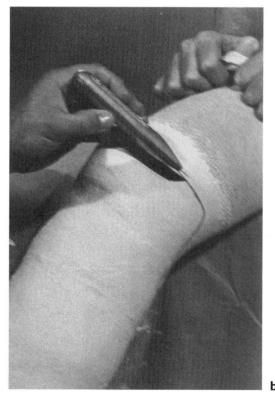

a   b

FIGURE 3.36. Once the plaster has hardened, the ultimate trim line is drawn. Superiorly, it goes slightly below the level of the proximal pole of the patella (**A**), laterally to the level of the hamstring muscles, and posteriorly to a point approximately 2 cm below a point opposite the tibial tubercle (**B**). With a sharp knife, the trimming is carried out.

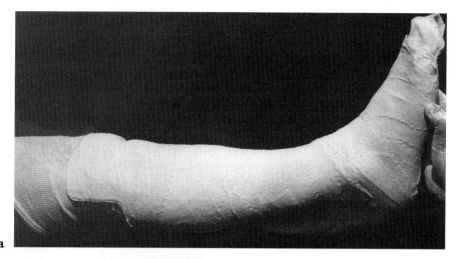

a

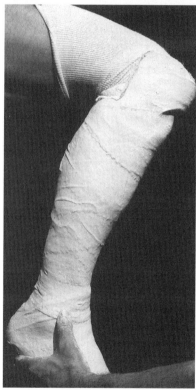

b

FIGURE 3.37. Upon completion of the trimming procedure, the knee should be able to flex and extend fully (**A and B**). Complete extension is not possible if the wrapping of plaster over the knee joints is conducted with the knee in flexion. Under these circumstances, the upper border of the plaster would cut into the patella as the joint was extended.

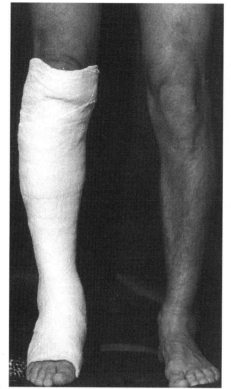

a

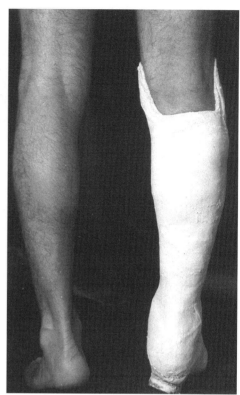

b

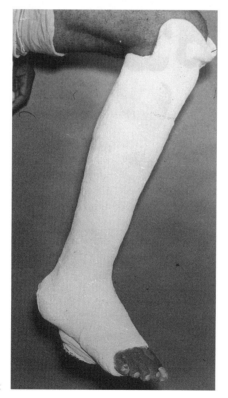

c

FIGURE 3.38. The completed functional cast shows the molding of the medial tibial condyle and medial distal tibial flare and the level of the anterior wall (**A**). Posteriorly are the closed contact of the "wings" of the plaster over the femoral condyles and the superior trim line below the popliteal skin line. A higher trimming would limit flexion of the knee and might irritate the hamstring tendons (**B**). Notice the placement of the walking heel, slightly in front of the axis of the tibia (**C**). During flexion of the knee, the firm contact between the "wings" of the plaster is lost, but it is regained during extension of the joint. It is during the stand (extension) phase of gait that the knee extends and therefore the time when the plaster assists in preventing rotary and angular deformities.

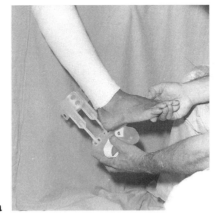
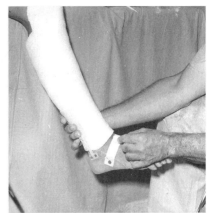

a

b

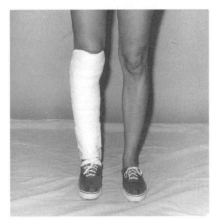
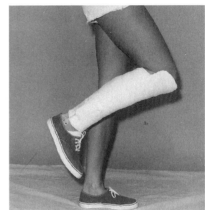

c, d

FIGURE 3.39. If the treating physician prefers the use of plaster for the fabrication of a brace, the leg segment of the below-the-knee functional cast is used. A plastic insert is placed under the patient's heel, which must be covered with a regular sock, not shown in these illustrations (**A**). The uprights of the insert are fastened to the underlying plaster with additional casting material (**B**). During assisted ambulation, the elastic plastic insert allows free motion of the foot and ankle while preventing rotary deformity (**C and D**).

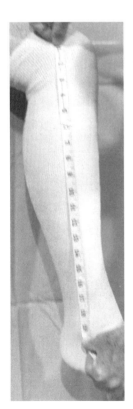

FIGURE 3.40. The functional brace may be custom-made using a variety of thermoplastic materials. The following photographs depict the use of Orthoplast (a synthetic balata). Measurements of the length of the leg are taken.

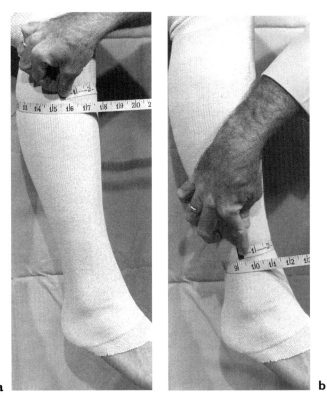

FIGURE 3.41.   The girth of the proximal (**A**) and distal ends of the leg are taken to select the appropriate prefabricated sheet of Orthoplast (**B**).

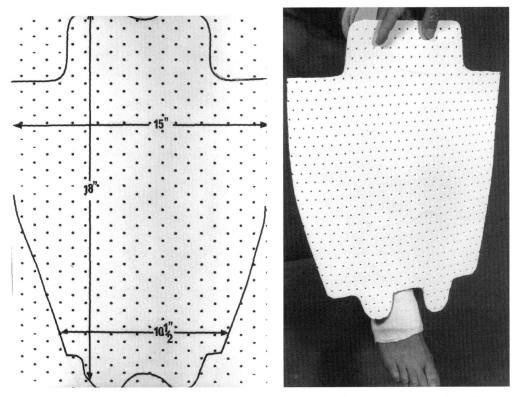

FIGURE 3.42.   Once the appropriate size sheet of Orthoplast is selected, its ultimate fit over the leg is estimated.

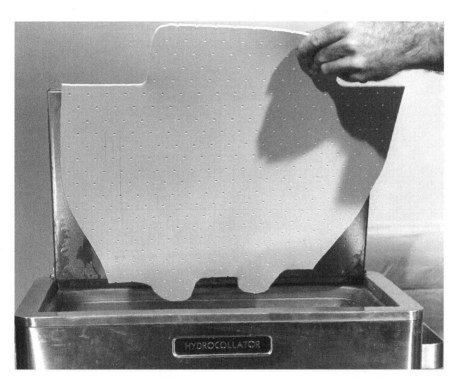

FIGURE 3.43. Then the sheet is dipped in hot water for approximately 5 minutes. The material softens and becomes malleable.

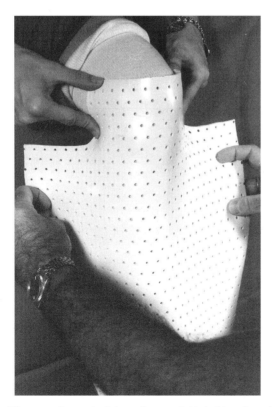

FIGURE 3.44. The superior end of the soft material is held against the patella and tibial condyles.

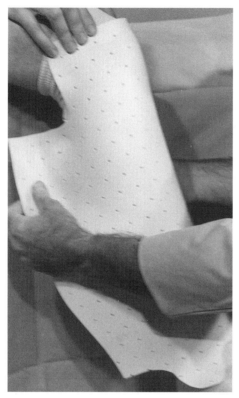
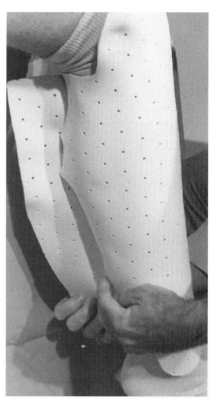

FIGURE 3.45. The material is then wrapped over the leg until its surfaces overlap. Because the material in the soft state is self-adhesive, care must be exercised to avoid premature contact between the yet-to-overlap surfaces.

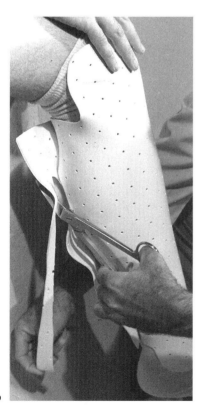
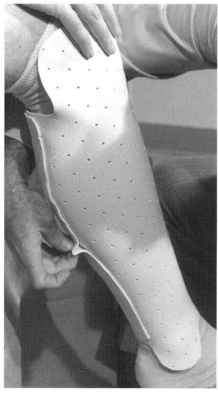

a, b

FIGURE 3.46. While holding the material firmly over the leg, gradual contact between its surfaces is obtained. Redundant material is removed with sharp scissors (**A and B**).

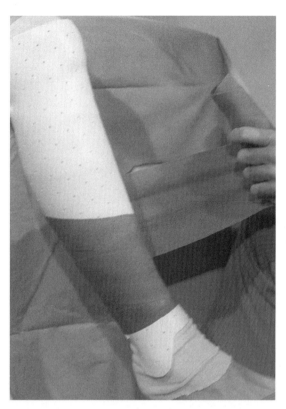 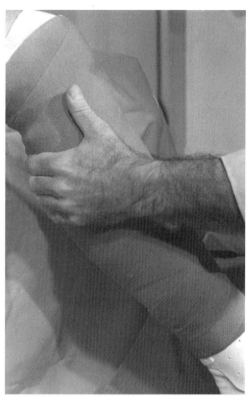

FIGURE 3.47.   An elastic bandage, saturated in cold water, is firmly wrapped over the entire Orthoplast material. Angular or rotary deformities are corrected at this time.

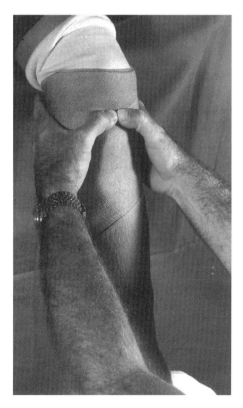

FIGURE 3.48.   Before the material begins to harden, the patellar tendon is gently indented, while avoiding excessive pressure over the area.

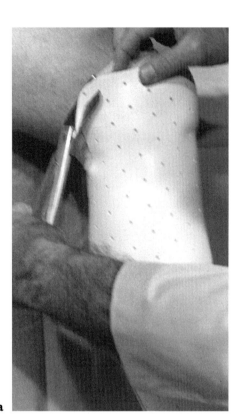
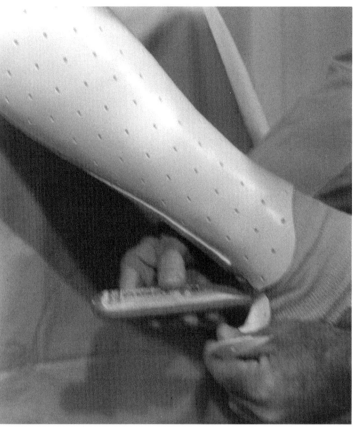

a   b

FIGURE 3.49. The proximal (**A**) and distal (**B**) ends of the plastic material are trimmed to eliminate areas of undesirable pressure over bony prominences and to permit unencumbered motion of the knee and ankle joints.

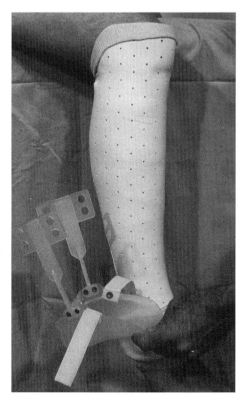

FIGURE 3.50. A plastic insert is then placed over the patient's heel.

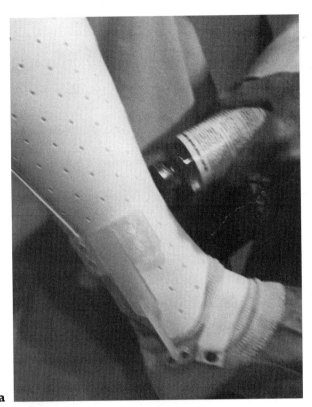

a

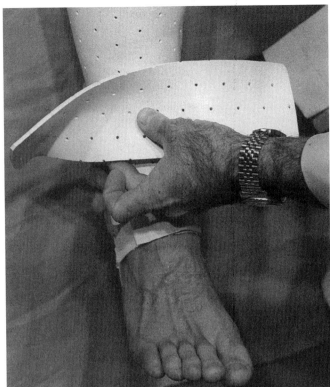

b

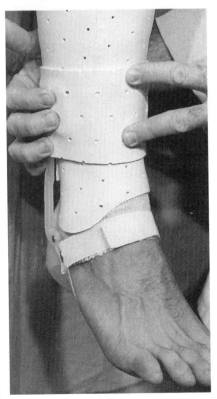

c

FIGURE 3.51. The uprights are held in place with heated straps of Orthoplast material. To enhance firm bonding between the surfaces of the plastic material, they are moistened with carbon tetrachloride before bringing them into contact with one another (**A–C**).

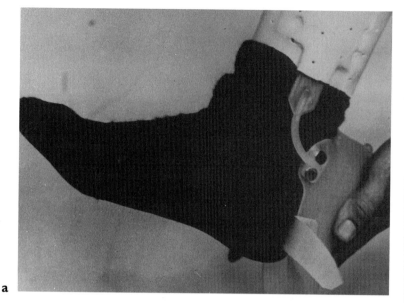

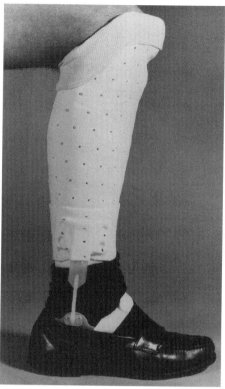

FIGURE 3.52. The patient is able to change socks and clean the foot by flexing the plastic insert posteriorly (**A**). A strap that holds the plastic liner in place prevents the distal slippage of the sleeve during the night when the shoe is removed (**B**).

a

b

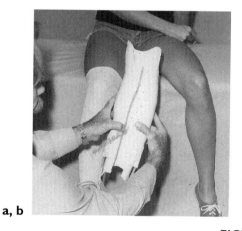

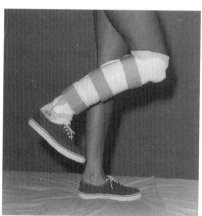

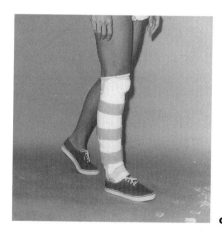

a, b

c

FIGURE 3.53. The Orthoplast brace can be made adjustable and removable by splitting it in the back with a power saw. Since the material is flexible, it can be removed from the leg and reapplied over it by spreading its margins apart (**A**). After attaching Velcro straps to the brace, adjustments can be easily made. It is highly desirable that the straps be frequently tightened to maintain compression of the soft tissue and enhance fracture stability (**B and C**).

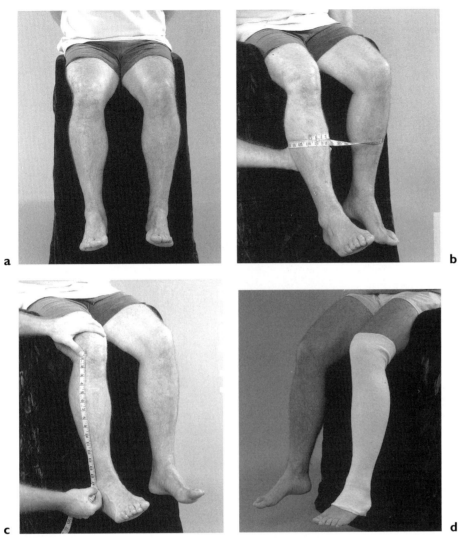

FIGURE 3.54.   Shown are the steps taken during the application of a prefabricated functional brace. With both legs exposed to ensure that the alignment of the injured extremity does not differ from the normal one (**A**), the girth and length of the distal leg are measured to select the appropriate brace size (**B and C**). A stockinet is rolled over the extremity extending to just above the knee joint (**D**).

deformity was not corrected at the time of brace application. The fracture healed with a deformity that could have been diagnosed either clinically or radiologically. When an anteroposterior radiograph of a normal tibia is taken with the toes pointing toward the ceiling, the leg is in slight internal rotation. In this position, the space between the tibia and the fibula is the greatest owing to the fact that the proximal tibiofibular joint is slightly posterior in reference to the tibia. If the leg is externally rotated, the fibula appears to hide behind the tibia. The greater the degree of internal rotation of the leg, the greater the distance between the two bones (Fig. 3.21). In this particular clinical case, the excessive external rotation of the distal fragment was not corrected; and when the brace was applied at a later date, the deformity was not appreciated, subjecting the patient to a permanent external rotation of the extremity (Fig. 3.21).

The patient was not aware of the abnormality, and only very close observation of his gait revealed to the examining surgeon the abnormal alignment. In instances when an external rotation abnormality has been present for several weeks in the cast, a prefabricated brace is not recommended if, during its application, the deformity cannot be corrected. It is best under this circumstance to reapply a cast after manual correction of the deformity is carried out or attempt the reduction during the molding of a custom-made brace.

The first step in the process of applying a prefabricated brace consists of measuring and recording the girth of the extremity at two different levels: over the most prominent portion of the calf and just above the ankle (Fig. 3.54A–C). The length of the limb is measured from the proximal pole of the patella to just below the lateral malleolus. The prefabricated brace was developed from measurements obtained in over 100 normal individuals. Three different sizes—small, medium, and large—were found to accommodate the overwhelming majority of people. The prefabricated brace was designed using the limbs of normal individuals as models, and therefore it does not accommodate major angular or rotary deformities.

Once the appropriate size of brace is chosen, the next step is to roll stockinet over the extremity, extending from the toes to just above the knee joint (Fig. 3.54D). Then the selected brace is slipped over the foot until it reaches the knee joint (Fig. 3.55). The patient's heel sits firmly on the plastic foot insert (Fig. 3.55). Once the brace is in place, the Velcro straps are fastened, from distally to proximally (Fig. 3.55). Once the initial tightening of the Velcro straps is done, the tightening must be performed again until the desirable even fit of the brace is obtained.

Upon completion of the bracing procedure, the patient should be able to fully extend and flex the knee (Fig. 3.56). If the limb has been stabilized in an above-the-knee cast for >2 weeks, it is not always possible to flex and extend the knee completely on the day of application of the brace. The surgeon should then observe carefully the proximal and distal ends of the brace to ascertain that it is not too long. If it is too long, the edge of the brace will impinge into the hamstring tendon or into the Achilles tendon. Ambulation should always begin with the aid of two crutches or a walker, and the degree of weight to be borne on the extremity should be minimal at first. It is increased gradually and according to the degree of symptoms produced by weight bearing. Under no circumstances should patients be encouraged to bear full weight on the injured extremity if there is pain. The use of only one crutch must begin only when weight bearing in this fashion is not accompanied with pain (Fig. 3.57).

It is best not to instruct patients on the technique of applying or removing the brace when the appliance is first donned. During the first week after the application of the brace, the patient should simply tighten the Velcro straps a couple of times a day to compensate for the decreased swelling that allows the brace to slip distally. It is highly advisable during these first few days to elevate the injured limb frequently and to exercise the knee and ankle joints. The combination of gradual, progressive weight-bearing ambulation and exercises of the ankle produces motion at the fracture site, enhancing, in this manner, osteogenesis.

During the first follow-up visit to the physician, the brace is removed, and the patient is instructed in the performance of the procedure. It is possible in most instances for patients to learn the technique of donning and doffing the brace and the application of a new stocking. The shoe is first removed (Fig. 3.58A). Then the Velcro straps are loosened (Fig. 3.58B), and the brace is slipped distally over the foot and ankle (Fig. 3.58C). Notice that the brace is made in a manner that prevents the straps from coming out of the buckles. This greatly facilitates the reapplication of the brace.

RESULTS

The orthopaedic literature is rich in reports regarding the use of functional bracing in the treatment of diaphyseal tibial fractures. Most reports indicate that under the appropriate circumstances and with adherence to accepted protocols, the clinical results obtained have been satisfactory. Every reporting author acknowledges the limitation of the system and finds surgical treatment to be the method of choice for a large percentage of fractures.

There is uniform agreement that the best indications for bracing of diaphyseal tibial fractures are those that are the result of low-energy trauma. Axially unstable fractures associated with initially unacceptable shortening are not good candidates for functional bracing as the corrected initial shortening is likely to recur after the introduction of weight bearing.

In this manual, we report only on our own results, which have been published in peer-reviewed orthopaedic journals (27–40). The most recent report was based on a series of 1,000 closed diaphyseal tibial fractures (39). The incidence of nonunion was 1.1%. Neither the age of the patient nor the location of the fracture influenced the speed of healing. In 95% of the fractures, the final shortening was <12 mm. The mean final shortening was 4.2 mm compared with the mean initial shortening of 4.25 mm.

The final angular deformity in any plane was <6 degrees in 90% of patients.

The presence of an intact fibula was a relative contraindication for functional bracing because angular deformity was more likely to occur. The intact fibula in oblique or comminuted fractures located in the proximal or distal thirds of the tibia is likely to create an unacceptable deformity and should not be braced early.

The acute cost of functional bracing was found to be significantly lower than that of intramedullary nailing. The estimated cost of treatment with intramedullary nailing was $6,811 compared with $2,781 for functional bracing. These figures do not include secondary treatment that may require a second or third hospitalization, such as nail removal.

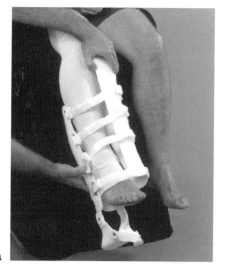

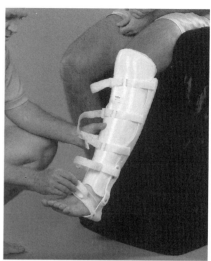

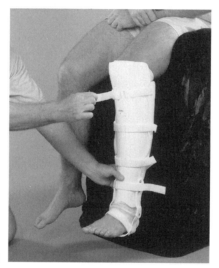

FIGURE 3.55. Once the appropriate brace is selected, it is slid over the patient's foot until it reaches the knee joint. The patient's heel should sit firmly over the plastic cuff (**A and B**). The Velcro straps are then tightened from distally to proximally (**C**).

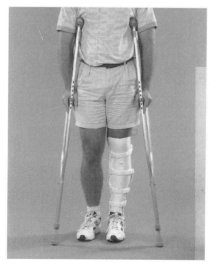

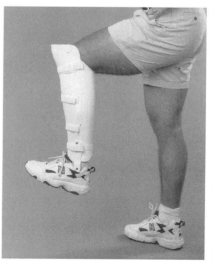

FIGURE 3.56. Upon completion of brace application, the patient may once again assume the erect position, always assisted with double external support. The knee should flex and extend fully (**A and B**). If the trimming lines of the brace limit flexion or extension of the knee or ankle, the excessive material can be removed with a pair of sharp scissors.

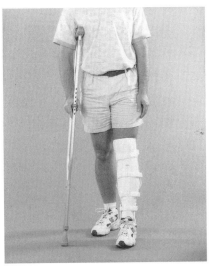
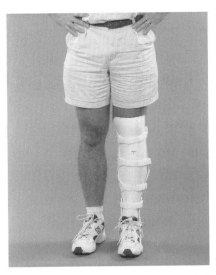

FIGURE 3.57. Upon subsidence of symptoms, the patient may graduate to ambulation, simply assisted with one crutch (**A**). Under no circumstances should patient be encouraged to ambulate without external support if weight bearing produces pain (**B**).

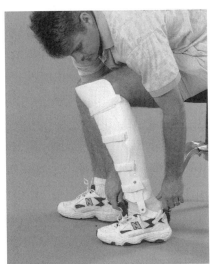
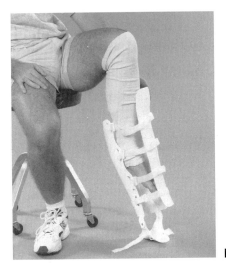

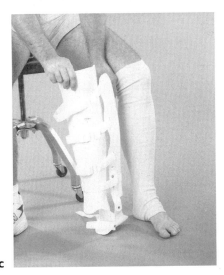

FIGURE 3.58. The patient should be able to temporarily remove the brace for hygienic purposes. The shoe is removed (**A**). The Velcro straps are loosened, and the brace is slid distally over the foot and ankle (**B and C**).

BASIC GUIDELINES FOR PHYSICIANS

DIAPHYSEAL TIBIAL FRACTURES

1. **Indications for functional bracing:** Indications include (a) primarily closed, axially unstable low-energy-produced fractures, such as oblique, spiral, comminuted, with <10 mm of initial shortening; (b) low-grade open fractures associated with minimal soft tissue damage and acceptable initial shortening; (c) axially stable fractures, that is, transverse fractures, providing a stable reduction is obtained; and (d) well-aligned fractures with a correctable <5 to 8 degrees of angular deformity.

2. **Contraindications:** Contraindications include (a) open fractures with severe soft tissue damage; (b) axially unstable fractures associated with unacceptable initial shortening; (c) closed and open fractures when acceptable alignment cannot be achieved (fractures with unacceptable initial shortening, if brought to length, might experience recurrence of shortening); (d) limbs with impaired sensation; and (e) oblique or comminuted fractures in the proximal or distal thirds with an intact fibula (these fractures might angulate into varus).

3. **How much shortening can be accepted:** Ten to 15 mm of shortening can be accepted; also, shortening in which the result of overriding fragments does not produce a limp or result in undesirable sequelae. Closed fractures experience, at the time of the initial injury, the final and total shortening.

4. **How much angular deformity can be accepted:** Angular deformities should be corrected. Five to 8 degrees of permanent angulation on any plane is usually acceptable as it is not readily recognized under visual inspection in many instances and does not lead to late arthritic changes. It is best to eliminate any angular deformity at the time of reduction and subsequent brace stabilization to minimize the risk of increased deformity.

5. **When to brace:** All tibial fractures should be initially stabilized in above-the-knee casts. Bracing should be carried out when acute swelling and pain have subsided. Most closed low-energy fractures permit bracing before the end of the second week after injury. Radiographic confirmation of acceptable fracture alignment is determined immediately after application of the brace. Frequent active exercises of the knee and ankle are encouraged.

6. **When to initiate ambulation:** Weight-bearing ambulation may begin as soon as the brace is applied, and its degree is dictated by the degree of symptoms. Two crutches must be used until all symptoms disappear. Mild discomfort can be expected during the first couple of weeks but should decrease gradually. Pain over bony prominences must be monitored carefully to ensure that pressure sores do not develop.

7. **Brace adjustment:** Braces are adjustable to maintain the necessary snugness of fit. The Velcro straps should be tightened frequently to compensate for the rapid disappearance of swelling. When the swelling stabilizes, adjustments are less frequent. At night, the shoe can be removed, but the dorsal strap must be in place.

8. **When to evaluate progress:** One week after the initial fit of the brace, progress should be evaluated. During that week, the patient is not allowed to remove the brace; only regular tightening of the straps is permitted. An x-ray film is obtained to confirm the maintenance of length and alignment of the fragments. At this time, the physician removes the brace to inspect the skin. The patient learns the technique of donning and doffing the brace for hygienic purposes. Subsequent visits should take place at approximately 4-week intervals.

BASIC GUIDELINES FOR PATIENTS

DIAPHYSEAL TIBIAL FRACTURES

1. **Prevention of swelling:** After application of the brace, it is common to see swelling of the foot develop. To reduce the swelling, the leg should be elevated frequently and the joint actively exercised. As time passes and the fracture heals, the amount of swelling decreases.

2. **Adjusting the brace:** Since the fractured leg is still swollen at the time of application of the brace, it is important that the Velcro straps of the brace be frequently tightened to accommodate changes in the girth of the extremity. During the first couple of weeks, frequent adjustments are encouraged. As the swelling is stabilized, the adjustments are needed less frequently. A snug brace is more comfortable than a loose one and ensures maintenance of good alignment of the fractured fragments.

3. **When to begin bearing weight on the fractured extremity:** In general, patients with tibial fractures treated with functional braces are encouraged to begin weight bearing as soon as the brace is applied. The amount of initial weight should be minimal and always assisted with two crutches or a walker. The degree of pain experienced at the site of the fracture should dictate the degree of weight to be borne. If a certain degree of weight bearing produces pain, it means that less weight is more appropriate. The amount of weight is increased slowly as the symptoms decrease.

4. **When to first remove the brace:** It is very likely that patients will not be allowed to remove the brace for hygienic purposes during the week after its application. At the end of the week, the patient will be instructed in the technique of temporary loosening of the brace, to make possible a change of stockinet and cleansing of the leg. This should not be done more than once a day. The shoe may be removed at night, but the dorsal Velcro strap must be snugly held in place to prevent distal displacement of the brace.

5. **Preventing pressure sores:** The sharp margins of the brace may produce excessive pressure over the skin. The discomfort and pain associated with that pressure, if not treated, will lead to painful skin sores. It is important that excessive pressure be prevented from the very outset. If the symptoms appear later, the treating physician must be notified.

6. **When to permanently discontinue the brace:** It is likely that the patient will be followed by the treating physician every 4 weeks, at which time new x-ray films will be obtained. Once the fracture has solidly healed, the brace will be discontinued. Under no circumstances should a patient ambulate without the brace if complete healing has not been documented. Failure to follow this instruction usually results in deformity of the leg. Most closed tibial fractures heal within 12 to 20 weeks.

7. **Shortening and angulation of the tibia:** Fractures treated without surgery and with the use of braces sometimes heal with a slight angulation and shortening. The average shortening in closed fractures of the tibia is <1 cm. This resulting discrepancy in the length of the legs does not produce a limp. A few degrees of angulation, <10 degrees, is rarely noticed under inspection. Scars from surgery are more likely to be noticed than a few degrees of angulation.

REFERENCES

1. Austin RT. Sarmiento tibial plaster: prospective study of 145 fractures. *Injury* 1981;13: 10.
2. Beach RB. Management of a tibial fracture using a patellar tendon bearing cast-brace. *Phys Ther* 1977;57:655.
3. Beard DJ, et al. Functional bracing: an alternative treatment for peri-articular fractures of the proximal tibia. *J Bone Joint Surg (Br)* 1985;67:145.
4. Brown PW. Early weight-bearing treatment of open fractures of the tibia. An end result of sixty-three cases. *J Bone Joint Surg (Am)* 1969;51:59.
5. Bruggemann H, Kujat R, Tscherne H. Funkionelle Frakturebehandlung nach Sarmiento an Unterschenkel,, Unterarm und Oberarm. *Orthopade* 1983;12:143.
6. Dehne E. Treatment of fractures of the tibial shaft. *Clin Orthop* 1969;66:159.
7. Delamarter R, Hohl M. The cast brace and tibial plateau fractures. *Clin Orthop* 1989; 242:26.
8. Ekkernkamp A, Kayser M, Althoff M. Knozept der Funktionellen Therapie am Beispiel des Frischen Geschlossenen Oberarmschaftbruches. *Zentralbl Chir* 1989;114:788.
9. Ekkernkamp A, Muhr G. Indikation und Technik der Funktionellen Knochenbruchbe-handlung Oper- und Unterarm. Unfallmed. Landesver. Gewerblich, GEW.BG, 1985.
10. Hardy AE. Ipsilateral fractures of the femoral and tibial diaphyses treated by cast-brace application. *J Bone Joint Surg (Br)* 1986;68:677.
11. Keating JF, Orfaly R, O'Brien P. Knee pain after tibial nailing. *J Orthop Trauma* 1997;11:10–13.
12. Kristensen KD, Kiaer T, Blicher J. No arthrosis of the ankle 20 years after malaligned tibial-shaft fracture. *Acta Orthop Scand* 1989;60:208.
13. Kujat R, Tscherne H. Indications and technique of functional fracture treatment with the Sarmiento brace. *Zentralbl Chir* 1984;109:1417.
14. Latta LL, Sarmiento A. Mechanical behavior of tibial fractures. In: *Symposium on trauma to the leg and its sequelae*. St. Louis: Mosby, 1981.
15. Lippert FG, Hirsch C. The three-dimensional measurement of tibial fracture motion by photogrammetry. *Clin Orthop* 1974;105:130.
16. Llinas A, McKellop H, Marshall J, et al. Healing and remodeling of articular incon-gruities in a rabbit fracture model. *J Bone Joint Surg (Am)* 1993;75:1508–1523.
17. Lovasz G, Llinas A, Benya P, et al. Effects of valgus tibial angulation on cartilage degen-eration in the rabbit knee. *J Orthop Res* 1995;13:846–853.
18. Lovasz G, Park SH, Ebramzadeh E, et al. Characteristics of degeneration in an unstable knee with a coronal surface step-off. *J Bone Joint Surg (Br)* 2001;82:428–436.
19. Lowrie IG, Reyes E, Meggitt BF. Functional recovery of tibial shaft fractures: fixed ver-sus hinged ankle cast brace. *J Bone Joint Surg (Br)* 1987;69:153.
20. McCollough NC, Vinsant JE, Sarmiento A. Functional fracture—bracing of long-bone fractures of the lower extremity in children. *J Bone Joint Surg (Am)* 1978;60:314.
21. McKellop HA, Sigholm G, Redfern FC, et al. The effect of simulated fracture-angulation of the tibia on cartilage pressures in the knee joint. *J Bone Joint Surg (Am)* 1991;73: 1382–1390.
22. Park S-H, O'Conner K, McKellop H, et al. The influence of active shearing compression motion on fracture healing. *J Bone Joint Surg (Am)* 1998;80:868–878.
23. Peter RE, Bachelin P, Fritschy D. Skiers' lower leg shaft fracture—outcome in 91 cases treated conservatively with Sarmiento's brace. *Am J Sports Med* 1988;16:486.
24. Ricciardi-Pollini PT, Falez F. The treatment of diaphyseal fractures by functional brac-ing: results in 36 cases. *Ital J Orthop Traumatol* 1985;11:199.
25. Rinaldi E, Marenghi P, Corradi M. The treatment of tibial fractures by elastic nailing and functional plaster cast. *Ital J Orthop Traumatol* 1987;13:173.
26. Rosa G, Savarese A, Chianca I, et al. Treatment of fractures of the lower limb with func-tional braces. *Ital J Orthop Traumatol* 1982;8:301.
27. Sarmiento A. Application of prosthetic principles to fracture care. *Spectator Lett* 1963.
28. Sarmiento A. A functional below-the-knee cast for tibial fractures. *J Bone Joint Surg (Am)* 1967;49:855.
29. Sarmiento A. A functional below-the-knee brace for tibial fractures. *J Bone Joint Surg (Am)* 1970;52:295.
30. Sarmiento A. Functional bracing of tibial and femoral shaft fractures. *Clin Orthop* 1972; 82:2.

31. Sarmiento A. A functional bracing of tibial fractures. *Clin Orthop* 1974;105:202.

32. Sarmiento A, Gerstein LM, Sobol PA, et al. Tibial shaft fractures treated with functional bracing. *J Bone Joint Surg (Br)* 1989;71:602.

33. Sarmiento A, Kinman PB, Latta LL. Fractures of the proximal tibia and tibial condyles: a clinical and laboratory comparative study. *Clin Orthop* 1979;145:136.

34. Sarmiento A, Latta LL. *The closed functional treatment of fractures*. Heidelberg: Springer-Verlag, 1981.

35. Sarmiento A, Latta LL. Functional bracing in management of tibial fractures: the intact fibula. In: *Symposium on trauma to the leg and its sequelae*. St. Louis: Mosby, 1981.

36. Sarmiento A, Latta LL. Functional fracture bracing. A review article. *J Am Acad Orthop Surg* 1999;7:66–78.

37. Sarmiento A, Latta LL, Zilioli A, et al. The role of soft tissues in stabilization of tibial fractures. *Clin Orthop* 1974;105:116.

38. Sarmiento A, McKellop H, Llinas A, et al. Effect of loading and fracture motion on diaphyseal tibial fractures. *J Orthop Res* 1996;14:80–84.

39. Sarmiento A, Sharpe MD, Ebramzadeh E, et al. Factors influencing the outcome of closed tibial fractures treated with functional bracing. *Clin Orthop* 1995;315:8–24.

40. Sarmiento A, Sobol PA, Sew-Hoy AL, et al. Prefabricated functional braces for the treatment of fractures of the tibial diaphysis. *J Bone Joint Surg (Am)* 1984;66:1328.

41. Sherman KP, Shakespeare DT, Nelson L, et al. A simple adjustable functional brace for tibial fractures. *Injury* 1986;17:15.

42. Suman RK. Orthoplast brace for treatment of tibial shaft fractures. *Injury* 1981;13:133.

43. Suman RK. Functional bracing in lower limb fractures. *Ital J Orthop Traumatol* 1983; 9:201.

44. Wagner KS, Tarr RR, Resnick C, et al. The effect of simulated tibial deformities on the ankle joint during the gait cycle. *Foot Ankle* 1984;5:131.

45. Zagorski JB, Latta LL, Finnieston AR. Comparative tibial fracture stability in casts, custom and pre-fabricated braces. *Orthop Trans* 1982;7:332.

46. Zagorski JB, Schenkman JH, Latta LL, et al. Pre-fabricated brace treatment of diaphyseal tibial fractures. *Orthop Trans* 1985;9:430.

47. Zych GA, Zagorski JB, Latta LL, et al. Modern concepts in functional fracture bracing—lower limb. In: *AAOS instructional course lectures, 26*. Chicago: American Academy of Orthopaedic Surgeons, 1987.

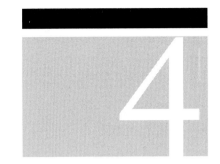

Other Indications for Functional Bracing

Rationale

Functional Bracing of Delayed Union and Nonunion of the Tibia

    Results

Functional Bracing of Colles' Fractures

    Results

Functional Bracing of Diaphyseal Femoral Fractures

    Results

Functional Bracing of Fractures of Both Bones of the Forearm

    Results

Basic Guidelines for Physicians

References

RATIONALE

In this manual, we have presented detailed descriptions of the rationale, indications, and technique of functional bracing of diaphyseal fractures of the humerus, ulna, and tibia. We selected those fractures because of comprehensive documented experiences that have assured them a place in the armamentarium of the orthopaedist. Though there are other fractures for which functional bracing is a sound therapeutic option, we have not given them extensive coverage. The decision to limit the extent of coverage was based on the facts that either the indications for functional bracing were limited, the clinical results thus far obtained were not sufficiently satisfactory to justify its promotion, or the technology necessary for its implementation was too complicated.

There are times when the treating physician, though aware of the greater value of surgical treatment in the management of a given patient, finds it necessary to apply a nonsurgical treatment in order to minimize risk and preserve the integrity of the injured limb. Other times, when the infrastructure of the facility where care is being provided lacks the sophistication necessary to ensure success with surgical treatments, conservative approaches are preferable. We have witnessed on many occasions disastrous complications following the surgical care of fractures that could have been managed by simple nonsurgical means. It appears that much too often, some surgeons believe that if the most modern surgical techniques are not used in all instances, their competency becomes subject to questioning.

Trends develop in the therapeutic approach to a variety of medical conditions. Often, the new trends prove to have improved the outcome of the treated conditions; other times, however, promising treatments are eventually abandoned, upon recognition that the initially suspected superiority of the new approaches was illusory. At this time, surgery has become the most popular approach to fractures in general. There is, however, not as yet sufficient evidence to justify the enthusiasm over a number of popular surgical treatments. For example, the "epidemic" of surgery in the treatment of Colles' fractures may come to an end if a close review of clinical (not radiologic) results demonstrates that the routine surgical reapproximation of fractured fragments does not bring about a better clinical outcome. The evidence might be that the indications for surgery are fewer than believed by some today, that the postoperative rehabilitation is longer, and that the overall cost of the surgical approach is unacceptably higher.

The entire world is struggling at this time with the fact that the cost of medical care continues to increase at a rather alarming pace. Though the etiology of this phenomenon is complex, there is little doubt that a major contributing factor is the use of new and expensive technology. Society is attempting to curtail the increasing medical cost by determining when expensive technology is necessary. Examples abound: The Colles' fracture may be used as a good one. If the clinical result from nonsurgical care of a certain types of Colles' fractures is equal to or better than that obtained from surgery, the former should be the recommended treatment. The use of surgical vertebral stabilization for the treatment of episodes of low back pain, in the absence of neurologic findings, without giving the patients the benefit of conservative measures, also serves as an appropriate example. The routine use of magnetic resonance imaging examinations for osteoarthritis of the hip raises the same question. The overwhelming majority of osteoarthritic conditions of the hip can be clearly diagnosed through simple radiologic techniques. Many other examples can be easily found—some of these in the care of fractures.

Unnecessary examinations and surgeries help to increase the cost of medical care. It behooves the medical profession to devote the utmost attention to seeing that the delivery of patient care is based not only on the true value of the various therapeutic options but on the cost of the treatments prescribed as well.

The fractures we are now briefly discussing in this chapter are tibial nonunions, Colles' fractures, diaphyseal femoral fractures, and fractures of both bones of the forearm. We have previously published preliminary experiences with functional bracing of those fractures. The appropriate references are included.

FUNCTIONAL BRACING OF DELAYED UNION AND NONUNION OF THE TIBIA

Most nonunions of the tibial diaphysis are currently managed with plate fixation, intramedullary nailing, or the Ilizarov method of distraction/impaction. Until now, the place of functional bracing in the care of this pathology has not been carefully explored. Our experiences have indicated that, under certain circumstances, the use of functional bracing brings about spontaneous healing of nonunions. The success rate in our reported 75 instances of delayed and nonunions of the tibia was 92%—a figure comparable with those reported in the literature from surgical treatments.

In most instances, the introduction of functional bracing is preceded by the performance of an ostectomy of the fibula at a level slightly above or below the nonunion site. A scientific explanation of the biology involved in the healing process is not fully available. We suspect that the ostectomy and the introduction of weight bearing constitute a new injury that brings about a biological response similar to that of an original injury. The newly created vascular, thermic, metabolic, chemical, and electrical factors create a stimulus to osteogenesis. The increased motion at the nonunion site works as the catalyst for the osteogenesis response. As soon as the acute symptoms that follow the ostectomy subside, the functional cast or brace is applied. In our series, the average time between the performance of the ostectomy and the application of the brace was about 1 week (Figs. 4.1 to 4.3).

An ostectomy is preferable to an osteotomy. A simple osteotomy may heal rapidly, depriving the nonunion site of the benefit of motion between the fragments. The ostectomy ensures a delay of healing of the fibula, even at the risk of developing nonunion of this bone. We found, in the review of our clinical material, that when a fibula nonunion developed, healing of the nonunited tibia was rather consistent (Figs. 4.4 to 4.6).

We have used this method in the care of tibial delayed unions and nonunions when the overall alignment of the tibia is acceptable or the angular deformity is of such a small degree that it can be corrected at the time of the fibular ostectomy. Failure to adhere to this prerequisite results in an increased degree of deformity (26,29).

Function and weight bearing are carried out according to the degree of symptoms. Most patients find themselves able to ambulate with the aid of one cane by the end of the fourth week. The healing process is slow. In some instances, several months are required before union is demonstrated. We have observed that the functional use of the extremity in the presence of motion of all joints favorably improves the condition of the bony and soft tissue structures in the disabled limb. We suspect that in the event the method proves unsuccessful, any subsequent surgery is performed through tissues in a better condition to promote healing.

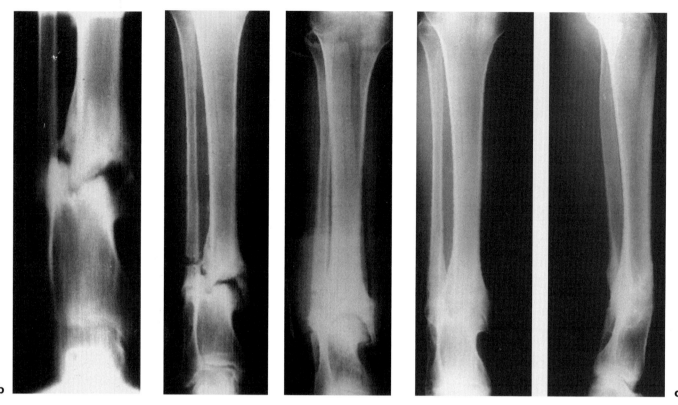

FIGURE 4.1. Nonunion of the tibia (**A**) was treated with fibular ostectomy followed by the application of a functional brace (**B**). The nonunion healed uneventfully (**C**).

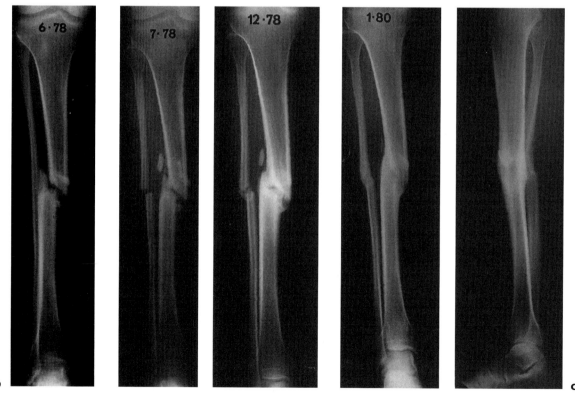

FIGURE 4.2. Nonunion of the tibia (**A**) was treated with fibular ostectomy followed by the application of a functional brace (**B**). The nonunion healed with minimal angular deformity (**C**).

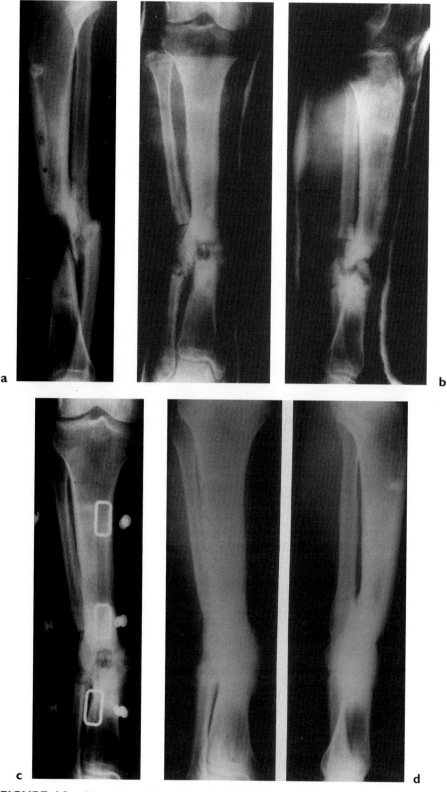

FIGURE 4.3.   Nonunion of the tibia, which had been subjected to several previous surgical procedures, is shown (**A**). A large fragment of the fibula was resected and placed over the tibial defect (**B**). A functional brace replaced the original above-the-knee cast (**C**). The nonunion healed uneventfully (**D**).

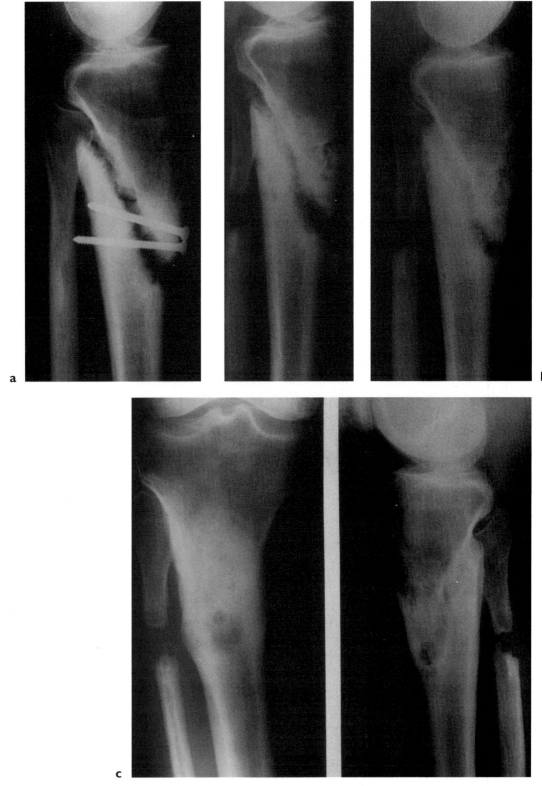

FIGURE 4.4.   Nonunion of the proximal tibia, which had been treated with fixation screws, is shown (**A**). A fibular ostectomy was performed and the leg stabilized in a below-the-knee functional brace (**B**). The nonunion healed, but the fibular defect persisted asymptomatically (**C**).

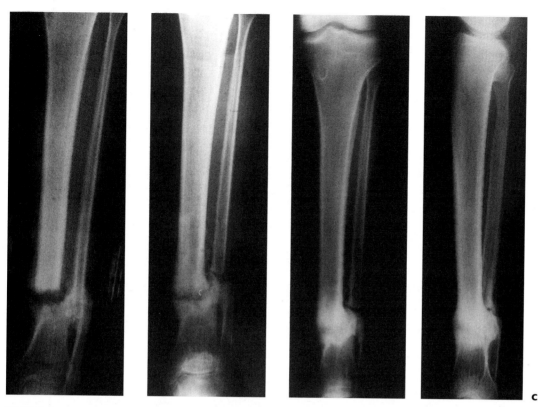

a, b   c

FIGURE 4.5.   Infected nonunion of the distal tibia (**A**) was treated with a fibular ostectomy and a functional brace (**B**). The nonunion healed, but a defect persisted between
the fibular fragments (**C**).

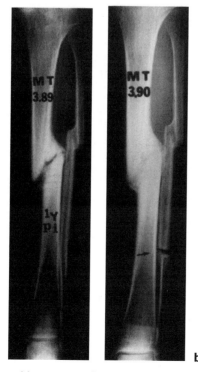

a   b

FIGURE 4.6.   One-year-old nonunion of the tibia (**A**) was treated with fibular ostectomy and the use of a functional fracture brace. The nonunion healed uneventfully. A
nonunion of the fibula persisted (**B**).

RESULTS

Our experiences with functional bracing of delayed union and nonunion of the tibia are limited to 73 patients. They were based on projects conducted at three different institutions: the University of Miami, the Fitzimus General Hospital in Denver, and the University of Southern California (29). Of these 73 patients, 22% had delayed union and 84.6% had nonunion.

The treatment consisted of only the application of a below-the-knee functional brace in 15% of the patients; an ostectomy of the fibula, followed by the application of a brace in 71.5% of the patients; and ostectomy of the fibula, bone grafting, and the application of a functional brace in 13.6% of the patients. The use of a functional brace was the common denominator for the three groups.

In the group of nonunions, 44 were classified as hypertrophic and 8 as atrophic.

Before the initiation of functional treatment, patients with delayed union had been disabled from 5 to 9 months, and patients with nonunion were disabled for >9 months.

FUNCTIONAL BRACING OF COLLES' FRACTURES

For many fractures of long and short bones of the skeleton, open reduction with internal fixation is currently the most popular treatment. This trend is partly supported by evidence that certain fractures do better and/or are rehabilitated faster when treated by surgical means. Intramedullary nailing of femoral shaft fractures is a very good example. There are, however, other subtler reasons for the popularity of surgery: Surgery is more convenient for surgeons, it is more prestigious for them, and it generates for them a much greater financial recompense.

The popularity of surgical approaches to fracture care is also based on the apparent obsession, on the part of recently trained surgeons, with the belief that restoration of anatomic length and alignment is synonymous with a perfect functional and aesthetic result. Needless to say, this is a flawed perception. Minor deviations from the normal are very well tolerated. For example, as much as 1 cm of posttraumatic shortening of a tibia or femur does not produce a limp or create an environment that leads to future degenerative disease in the joints above and below the fracture. Similarly, minor angular or rotary deformities are not harmful to the adjacent joint (15–17,35).

Though good results in the care of Colles' fractures have been reported with the use of plate fixation and/or external fixation, and the beneficial place for these two modalities is well established, their use must be limited to those fractures not likely to respond well to equally effective nonsurgical methods of treatment. Plate fixation may be associated with infection, severe adhesion of soft tissues, damage to peripheral nerves, and possible additional damage to the injured articular fracture. The cost of care from plate fixation is higher, rehabilitation is required for a longer period of time, and removal of the implant is often necessary.

External fixation has also rendered good results in a number of Colles' fractures. The system is not a panacea, any more than functional bracing and plating are. Complications from its use are frequently reported. Pin tract infection is a very common accompanying complication. Limitation of motion of the wrist and fingers is also a common sequela that requires prolonged and expensive rehabilitation measures.

The increasing interest in surgical approaches to Colles' fractures is due, to a great extent, to the mistaken belief that restoration of length and congruity is essential for the attainment of a good result. There is ample evidence in the literature indicating that long-lasting good clinical results can be obtained in the presence of radiologically identified angular deformity and incongruity.

Of great importance in the assessment of results from the various treatment modalities is the recognition that the articular cartilage can be permanently damaged at the time of the injury, particularly if the injury was of the impaction type. Therefore, the surgical reapproximation of articular cartilage that is permanently damaged does not alter the ultimate prognosis. Arthritic changes are frequently seen in radiographs of healed Colles' fractures that were treated by closed or open methods. These arthritic changes are often asymptomatic and constitute simply an irrelevant radiologic finding.

Attempts to restore anatomical congruity of comminuted intraarticular fractures are not always successful. The final radiographs may show improvement, but a residual incongruity is frequently left behind.

Functional bracing provides clinically successful results in the majority of Colles' fractures. However, its place does not extend to all types of fractures. Comminuted Colles' fractures that have a dislocation of the distal radioulnar joint have a ready tendency to experience a recurrence of the original deformity in spite of a successful closed reduction (2,24,31,32,34). This pattern suggests that the stability of the distal radioulnar joint is the single most important prognostic feature in Colles' fractures. Mild incongruity per se is not the problem with intraarticular fractures; instability is the real culprit. Our laboratory investigations have documented this important point (15,17). Functional bracing should be reserved for those fractures with intact radioulnar joints and especially for the ones where the distal radial fracture is not intraarticular and/or comminuted.

Functional bracing should never be the initial treatment. The initial swelling precludes the application of a snug cast. The brace is applied a few days after the initial insult, when the acute symptoms have subsided and the swelling has decreased. The fracture, once reduced, should be stabilized with the forearm in a relaxed attitude of supination (Fig. 4.7). In this manner, the harmful action of the brachioradialis muscle is partially eliminated (24) (Figs. 4.8 and 4.9). The position of relaxed supination not only decreases the deforming force created by the brachioradialis muscle but also assists in other ways: (a) Flexion of the fingers and wrist is carried out with greater ease, when compared with pronation. (b) The radioulnar joint is more stable in supination. (c) Radiologic evaluation of the position of the fractured fragments is best conducted in supination. (d) Recognition of a scapholunate subluxation is more easily made with the forearm in supination. (e) Spontaneous improvement of loss of forearm motion takes place faster when the position of forearm stabilization is that of supination (Figs. 4.10 to 4.12).

Most activities of daily living require forearm pronation. Patients find themselves unconsciously forcing the forearm into pronation. As supination is required for fewer activities, a permanent limitation of supination is more likely to occur. If the forearm loses the last few degrees of pronation, this limitation is readily and inconspicuously compensated with a combined motion of shoulder flexion, abduction, and internal rotation—a mechanism similar to the one used by amputees who lack pronation and supination of the forearm. A similar inconspicuous mechanism does not exist to compensate for lack of supination.

The following example of a distal, extraarticular, not associated with a dislocation of the distal radioulnar joint, where a stable reduction was obtained

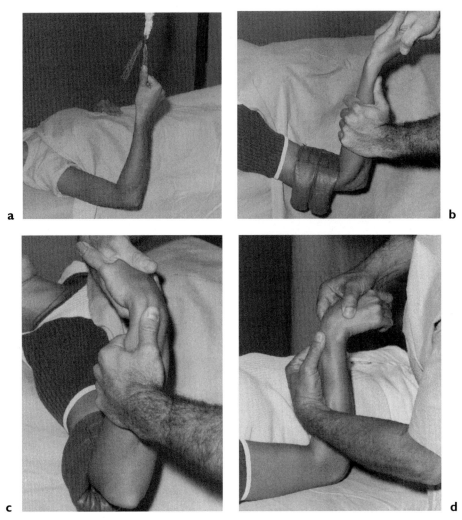

FIGURE 4.7. Before manipulating a Colles' fracture, it is useful to apply traction using "Chinese fingertraps" for a few minutes to assist in disengaging the bony fragments and to minimize the trauma of manual reduction (**A**). The traction should not exceed more than 5 to 7 lb and should not be held for more than 5 minutes. Then, the deformity is forcefully increased (**B**). The next step consists of correcting the dorsal angulation of the distal radial fragment (**C**). The forearm is then pronated, and pressure is applied over the lateral aspect of the distal radius to correct its radial deviation (**D**). Rotating the forearm assists in confirming the stability of the radioulnar joint, which is more stable in supination.

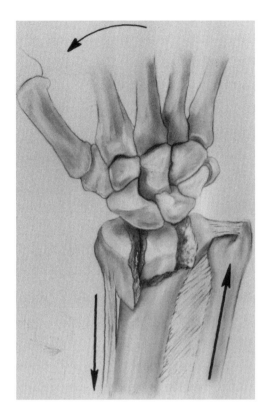

FIGURE 4.8. Schematic representation of comminuted Colles' fracture associated with dislocation of the distal radioulnar joint is presented. This type of fracture should not be braced because of the likely recurrence of the dislocation.

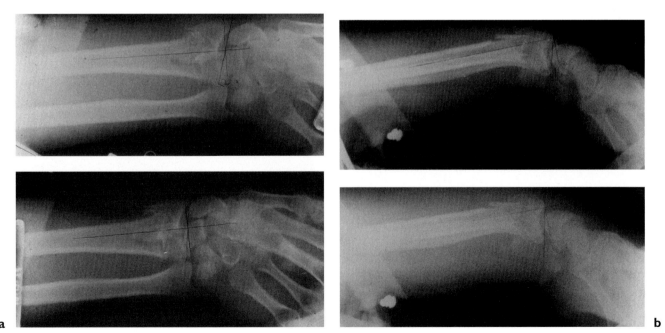

a   b

FIGURE 4.9. Anteroposterior radiographs of a reduced Colles' fracture are shown, before electrical stimulation of the brachioradialis muscle (**A, top**) and after electrical stimulation (**A, bottom**). Lateral radiographs taken during the electrical stimulation exercise are also presented (**B**). Notice that the electrical stimulation of the brachioradialis muscle produced a partial recurrence of dorsal and radial deviation.

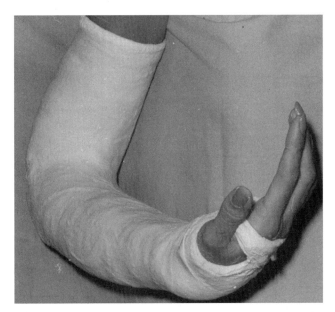

FIGURE 4.10.   Upon completion of the manipulative reduction, the forearm should be held in a relaxed attitude of supination and the wrist in slight flexion and ulnar deviation. All fingers should be free to function.

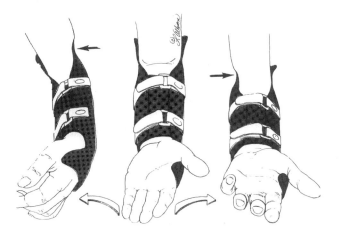

FIGURE 4.11.   The initial cast may be replaced at a later date with a functional brace. Schematic drawing of the functional brace used in the treatment of certain Colles' fractures is shown. Notice that palmar flexion is possible, while dorsiflexion is prevented by the brace. Radial deviation and pronosupination are also prevented by the brace.

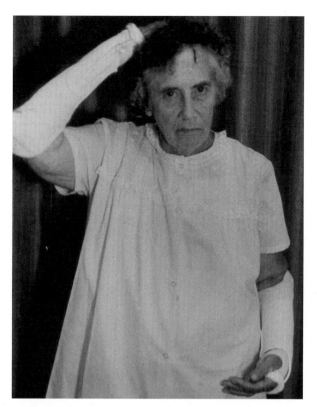

FIGURE 4.12.   A patient with bilateral Colles' fractures demonstrates the function of her upper extremities.

and maintained in the brace (Figs. 4.13 and 4.14). Extraarticular fractures, without associated dislocation of the distal radioulnar joint, that are reduced and rendered stable can be successfully treated with functional braces (Fig. 4.15).

RESULTS

The nonsurgical treatment of Colles' fractures still remains the treatment of choice in the vast majority of instances. However, this is true only for fractures that are extraarticular for which a closed manipulation renders a stable reduction, for those without dislocation of the distal radioulnar joint, and for intraarticular fractures with intact radioulnar joints, where an adequate restoration of congruity can be achieved by closed reduction (30,31).

After gaining experience with functional bracing of Colles' fractures treated with the forearm in a relaxed attitude of supination (31,32,38,39), we carefully evaluated our results and compared the outcome of those fractures treated in supination versus those treated in pronation.

One hundred fifty-six patients were treated and the results reported. Approximately one half of the fractures were immobilized in pronation and the other half in supination. One hundred four patients were seen at follow-up. The average length of follow-up was 15 weeks.

The braces were applied on an average of 7 days after the initial reduction and stabilization in a cast that immobilized the elbow and wrist joints. There was no significant difference in the period of immobilization between the pronation and supination groups. In the groups of minimally displaced fractures (whether intraarticular or extraarticular), there was no significant change in position of the fracture, from the time of injury to the last follow-up, regardless of whether braced in pronation or supination.

In the group of displaced extraarticular fractures, only one (8%) patient treated in supination lost radial length, while seven (39%) patients treated in pronation showed at least 2 mm of shortening. None of the supination-treated patients experienced any further loss of volar tilt once braced. However, three (17%) patients in the pronation category had further dorsal angulation of at least 2 degrees. There was no appreciable difference between the groups in regards to radial deviation.

Patients with intraarticular displaced fractures showed no difference with respect to radial displacement. However, the overall results in the pronation group were inferior to those in the supination group. After bracing in supination, 1 (5%) patient lost 2 degrees of dorsal tilt, whereas 10 (50%) patients in the pronation group angulated ≥2 degrees while in the brace. Similarly, 10 (50%) patients in the pronation-braced group continued to lose ≥2 mm of length. Only three (15%) patients braced in supination demonstrated shortening.

Incongruity is instinctively considered by many as a cause of posttraumatic osteoarthritis. However, mild incongruity is readily tolerated. We have demonstrated this fact in animal studies (15–17), and others have drawn the same conclusion from clinical experiences. Frykman (6), for example, reported a 19% rate of osteoarthritis, which he acknowledged was "frequently asymptomatic." Smail (33) reported on 41 patients followed between 5 and 6 years after fracture. Ten had x-ray changes of osteoarthritis, but only three had symptoms.

Instability in the presence of incongruity is probably a factor that leads to cartilage degeneration. We demonstrated that articular incongruities that experience spontaneous improvement and remain free of osteoarthritic changes develop degenerative changes when the joint is simultaneously rendered unstable (16,17).

We have critically reviewed our results with functional bracing of Colles' fractures and have also studied the results obtained by others using plate fixation and external fixator. We have come to the conclusion that surgery does not necessarily render better results than nonsurgical functional approaches. This conclusion does not negate the facts that a number of Colles' fractures are best treated by surgical means and that the use of bracing in those instances is inappropriate.

However, to use the surgical approach in the management of all Colles' fractures, simply because of the mistaken belief that anatomical reduction gives better results, is also inappropriate.

FUNCTIONAL BRACING OF DIAPHYSEAL FEMORAL FRACTURES

At this time, the vast majority of femoral shaft fractures are successfully treated by means of intramedullary nailing. The introduction of the concept of interlocking nails has made possible the surgical treatment of proximal and distal diaphyseal fractures, which the noninterlocking nail does not effectively manage. However, the technology of the interlocking nail is not available in all parts of the world to make its implementation safe. There are times when surgical fixation is not technically possible or when individual patient circumstances preclude the surgical approach. The medical condition of the patient might contraindicate surgery, and certain open fractures not seen promptly by the trained surgeon are likely to develop major complications when surgically violated.

Experiences with femoral fracture bracing have demonstrated that diaphyseal fractures above the middle third of the bone have a tendency to angulate into varus (1,3,4,5,7,8,10,11,13,14,18,19,20,23,25,29,36,37). Satisfactory results are frequently obtained when the method is used in fractures located in the distal third of the bone and the brace is applied after intrinsic stability at the fracture site has taken place (8–10,25,29) (Figs. 4.16 to 4.19) However, the method is expensive because of the required hospitalization until intrinsic stability of the fracture is demonstrated. Union is rather consistently achieved, the final angular deformity is usually within acceptable degrees, and the ultimate range of motion of the adjacent joints is comparable with that obtained with surgical management (25,29).

Basically, the indications for functional bracing are limited. The system should be reserved for special fractures and circumstances. It is a rewarding method of treatment in the care of fractures located distal to the femoral isthmus and practical in environments lacking modern surgical facilities.

The femoral functional brace may be fabricated using plaster of Paris or Orthoplast material (Johnson and Johnson). In this manual, we illustrate only the Orthoplast technique.

After the appropriate period of stabilization in traction, the brace may be applied. The period of bed confinement is determined by the severity of the injury, the degree of initial shortening and deformity, and other associated conditions. Fractures with significant shortening at the time of the initial insult heal more slowly than those with less initial shortening. Release of the traction before intrinsic stability develops at the fracture site results in a recurrence of shortening and angulation. Regardless of the time of stabilization required for the development of intrinsic stability, it is of the greatest importance to carry out passive exercises to the knee joint. A balanced suspension type of traction allows the patient to carry out the knee flexion and extension exercises on a frequent basis.

At the time of application of the brace, the patient must be in the supine position. An appropriate-size sheet of Orthoplast is selected. It should cover the entire length of the femur. Once it is dipped in warm water and made pliable, it is then wrapped over the thigh (Fig. 4.20A). The material is then firmly wrapped with an elastic bandage, which has been previously saturated in cold water (Fig. 4.20B). As the material hardens, the entire femur, especially the femoral condyles, is molded (Fig. 4.20C). The metallic joint is then attached to the brace, and the functional brace is completed according to traditional orthotic principles (Fig. 4.21).

RESULTS

Our personal experiences with functional bracing of femoral fractures took place in the days preceding the development of interlocking femoral nailing. The intramedullary femoral nail was being used exclusively for diaphyseal fractures, as it was felt that metaphyseal fractures treated in that manner were likely to fail to remain appropriately aligned. Our series with functional bracing, however, included a number of diaphyseal fractures because they were either segmental, comminuted, or, for a variety of reasons, considered to be unsuitable for intramedullary fixation. In addition, one must keep in mind that in the 1960s and 1970s, closed nailing had not been yet popularized in the United States.

Our documented experiences with femoral fracture bracing consisted of 245 patients (25,29). The patients' age ranged from 16 to 98 years. Eighty per-

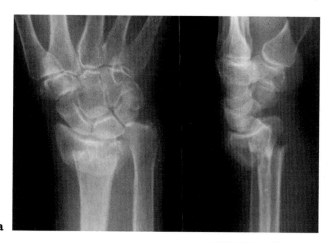
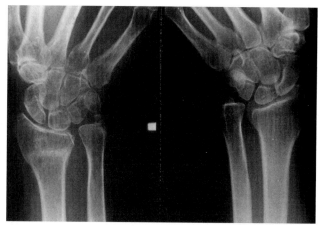

a   b

FIGURE 4.13. Extraarticular Colles' fracture was treated with a functional brace. Notice that the radioulnar joint is subluxated (**A**). This feature is frequently a contraindication of functional bracing if the reduction of the radial fracture does not render the joint stable. The fracture healed with a subluxated radioulnar joint but without associated symptoms (**B**).

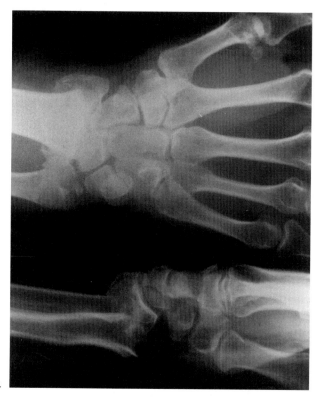
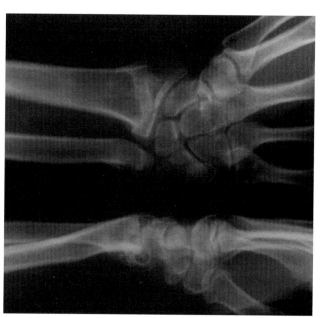

a   b

FIGURE 4.14. Extraarticular Colles' fracture with an associated fracture of the distal ulna is presented (**A**). The fracture was treated with a functional brace with a resulting minimal deformity (**B**).

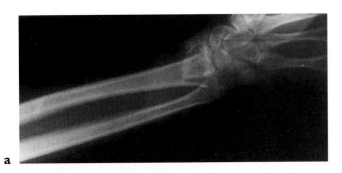

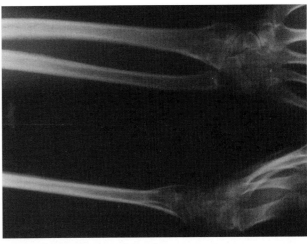

FIGURE 4.15. Intraarticular Colles' fracture (**A**), once reduced, became very stable. The fracture was then treated in a functional cast. The functional and anatomical results were satisfactory (**B**).

FIGURE 4.16. Comminuted fracture of the distal femur was produced by a low-velocity projectile. The fracture was treated with a functional femoral brace after 3 weeks of stabilization in balanced traction/suspension (**A**). The fracture healed with acceptable functional and cosmetic results (**B**).

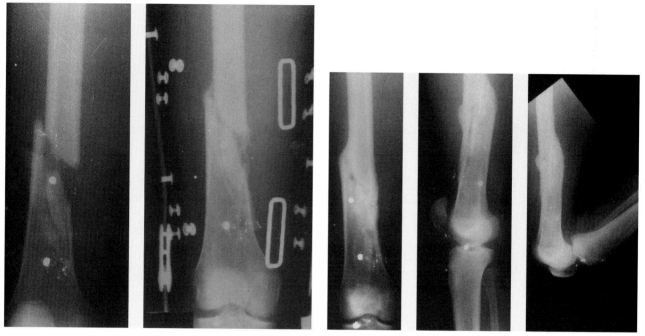

a   b

FIGURE 4.17.   Mildly comminuted fracture of the distal femur was the result of a bullet wound. A brace was applied after 4 weeks of stabilization in functional traction (**A**). The fracture healed with good alignment of the fragments and function of the knee joint (**B**).

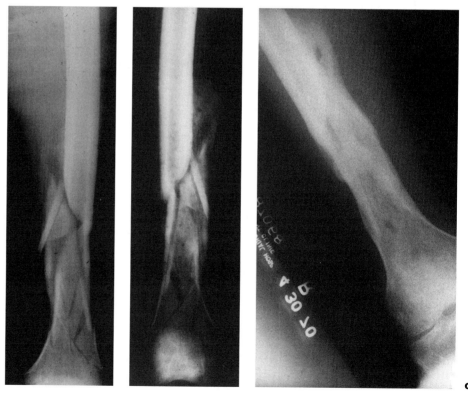

a, b   c

FIGURE 4.18.   Closed comminuted fracture of the distal femur was treated in a functional brace, after approximately 3 weeks in balanced traction (**A**). Progressive healing took place in the brace (**B**), and the fracture healed uneventfully (**C**).

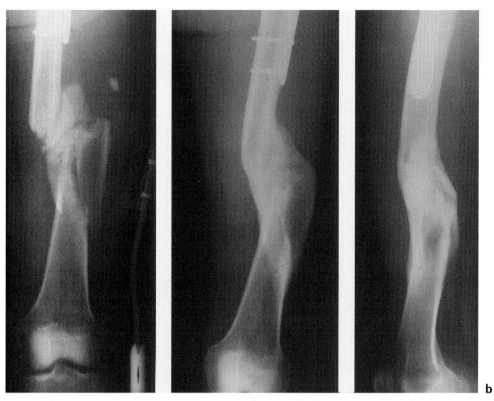

a   b

FIGURE 4.19.   Comminuted fracture of the distal third of the femur was treated with a functional brace, following 4 weeks of stabilization in balanced traction (**A**). The fracture healed with acceptable length and alignment (**B**).

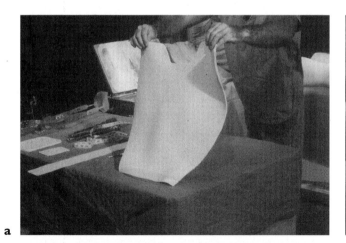

a

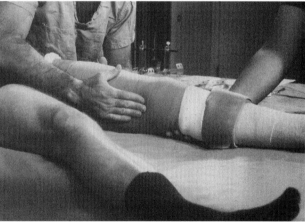

c

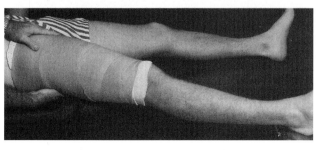

b

FIGURE 4.20.   Steps taken during the fabrication of an Orthoplast femoral fracture bracing: A sheet of Orthoplast, long enough to cover the entire thigh, is selected and dipped in hot water for approximately 5 minutes. This procedure makes the material soft and pliable (see Chapter 3) (**A**). The material is wrapped around the thigh and then firmly covered with an elastic bandage that has been previously saturated in cold water. The low temperature of the water expedites the hardening of the plastic material (**B**). During the setting process, the thigh is molded in a manner that attempts to achieve the most desirable points of pressure (**C**).

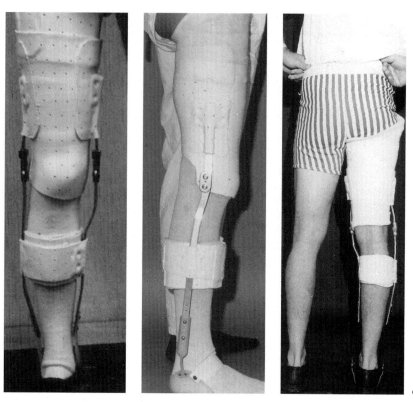

a, b   c

FIGURE 4.21. The metallic knee joint is attached to the brace and held in place with strips of Orthoplast. Upon completion of the bracing procedure, the brace should fit comfortably. There should be room for full range of motion of the hip, knee, and ankle joints (**A–C**).

cent of the fractures were closed and 20% were open. Of these, 7.3% were located in the proximal third of the humerus, 53.8% in the middle third, 35.5% in the distal third, and 3.2% were segmental (25,29).

Thirty-nine patients had associated major fractures. Forty-one (16.7%) were transverse, 31 (12.6%) were short oblique, 46 (18.7%) were spiral, 110 (48.5%) were comminuted, and 8 (3.2%) were segmental.

The average time elapsed between the onset of disability and the day of application of the brace was 5 weeks, with a median of 4.5 weeks and modes of 4, 6, and 8 weeks. The overall time in a brace was 9 weeks.

Residual angulation was measured by conventional means. Among the 18 fractures located in the proximal third of the femur, 55% had >10 degrees of varus. Of the 132 fractures in the middle third, 17% had >10 degrees of varus angulation and 4% >10 degrees of valgus angulation. Among the 87 fractures located in the distal third of the femur, 6% had >10 degrees of varus angulation and 2% >10 degrees of valgus angulation.

Final shortening of the injured extremity in the patients with fractures located in the proximal third of the femur had a median of 3 cm, those in the middle third 1.5 cm, those in the distal third 1.5 cm, and the segmental ones 2 cm.

Of the 216 whose range of motion of the knee was recorded, 154 (71%) patients regained full range of motion; 36 (16.6%) patients lost <10% of flexion, 16 (7.4%) patients lost <15 degrees of flexion, 6 (2.7%) lost <20% of flexion, and 4 (1.8%) lost <25 degrees of flexion.

FUNCTIONAL BRACING OF FRACTURES OF BOTH BONES OF THE FOREARM

Plating is currently the most common method of treatment of fractures of both bones of the forearm. The technique is simple, the incidence of complications is low, and the final clinical outcome is satisfactory in most instances. However, the method may result in a higher incidence of nonunion, the development of synostosis and infection, and subsequent refracture. To a lesser extent, the same applies to intramedullary nailing. It is likely that refinement in the use of imaging technology will increase the successful use of nailing.

Plating gained popularity upon recognition of the difficulties encountered in reducing and maintaining reduction in some instances. However, little attention has been given to the fact that the forearm tolerates well minor deviations from the normal. Five to 10 degrees of angulation or 5 to 10 degrees of malrotation is likely to go unnoticed from the cosmetic and functional points of view (27–29,35). Reports from China and other Eastern countries have eloquently demonstrated the excellent results that can be obtained with the use of stabilizing bamboo splints.

The widespread practice of surgically approaching fractures in all instances is due to the mistaken perception that anatomical reduction is essential for the attainment of good results. What we have failed to recognize is that the efforts to achieve anatomical reduction are frequently responsible for the subsequent loss of reduction. The acceptance of overriding fragments, in the presence of acceptable alignment, results in minimal or no permanent loss of pronosupination (Figs. 4.22 and 4.23).

More recently, there has been an effort to popularize the use of plating and nailing in children over the age of 6. Reports have suggested a low incidence of complications. Though we recognize that there are situations when internal fixation of forearm fractures in growing children is the treatment of choice, it is difficult for us to accept the fact that all these fractures should be treated surgically. There are complications from anesthesia and surgery, which, though rare, may be of a serious nature. Furthermore, plates produce a callus of an inferior nature, and their removal is often necessary. A high incidence of refracture has been reported in the literature.

Successful plating is usually associated with a residual mild, permanent limitation of pronosupination. This loss is not usually recognized by the patients and can be demonstrated only with critical methods designed to precisely measure degrees of motion. If the loss of motion is limited to pronation, patients compensate very inconspicuously by internally rotating the shoulder joint (28). This is the same mechanism used by amputees whose terminal device does not permit rotation of the forearm. There is not, however, a comparable inconspicuous mechanism for the lack of supination.

The loss of pronosupination that our patients with fractures of both bones of the forearm demonstrated upon completion of healing was minimal, despite the fact that radiographs had demonstrated angular deformities (27–29). Rotary deformities, if they are only of a few degrees, are not associated with detectable functional impairment. Our laboratory studies demonstrated that for every degree of malrotation, there is a resultant loss of 1 degree of pronosupination (35). When we compared the final loss of pronosupination of our patients with the loss of that motion in cadavers with artificially created identical deformities, we discovered that humans experienced less limitation of motion than found in cadavers (28).

Our experience with functional casting and bracing of fractures of both bones of the forearm has indicated that transverse fractures, once reduced and stabilized in a cast, are likely to suffer angulation, particularly if the initial injury produced major degrees of swelling (27–29). Upon the subsidence of swelling, the stabilizing cast loses its efficacy and angular deformity develops. This complication is more likely to take place if one of the bones sustains a transverse fracture and the other bone sustains an oblique fracture. In this instance, the angulation is in the direction of the oblique fracture. Therefore, transverse displaced fractures of both bones, particularly those located close to the wrist or elbow, are best treated with plate osteosynthesis.

Closed forearm fractures experience, at the time of the initial injury, the total and final amount of shortening. This is similar to that of closed tibial fractures. Closed fractures demonstrate, in the vast majority of instances, a degree of shortening that is minimal and inconsequential. This shortening, in the absence of major angular or rotary malalignment, produces no or minimal functional limitation of motion, a limitation comparable with that seen after successful plating (7,18,19).

The fractures of both bones of the forearm most amenable to closed functional casting or bracing are the ones where the fractures are oblique or comminuted. The shortening remains essentially unchanged, and the alignment of the fragments is usually maintained (Figs. 4.22 and 4.23).

Functional casting or bracing is not indicated as the initial treatment. The swelling that results from the injury precludes the firm compression of the soft tissues that is necessary for success after bracing. The functional cast or brace can be applied only after a period of stabilization of the fracture in an above-the-elbow cast that holds the forearm in a relaxed position of supination (Fig. 4.24). Once the brace is applied with the elbow in the same position of supination, the wrist is free to move in volar and dorsal directions, and the elbow can be flexed fully, but its extension is limited in the last 20 to 25 degrees. Pronation and supination are not possible (Fig. 4.25).

If Orthoplast material is not available, plaster of Paris may be used. The principles of application remain the same. The forearm must be held in a relaxed attitude of supination throughout the entire procedure, while the extremity is suspended using approximately 5 lb of traction, applied though Chinese fingertraps. The anterior and posterior surfaces of the forearm are firmly compressed to separate the two bones as much as possible (Figs. 4.24E and 4.26A). The plaster of Paris, which incorporates the elbow being held in approximately 45 degrees of flexion, is then trimmed to make possible eventual flexion of the elbow. Posteriorly, the trimming should be as high as possible to limit flexion of the elbow. The supracondylar regions are molded over the distal humerus, avoiding, however, excessive pressure over neurovascular structures (Fig. 4.26).

RESULTS

Our published reports dealing with functional bracing of both bones of the forearm consisted of only 39 patients (27,29). One patient (2.5%) had the fractures located in the proximal third of the forearm. Twenty-eight (71.9%) patients had the fractures in the middle third, and 10 (25.6%) patients had them located in the distal third. Losses of <18% were noted for distal and middle third fractures with ≤10 degrees of total angular deformity. We do not consider this loss to be clinically important (27–29,35). We strongly suspect, based on clinical observations, that patients who have successful plating procedures performed in the care of fractures of both bones of the forearm experience a comparable loss of pronosupination.

There were no nonunions in this small group.

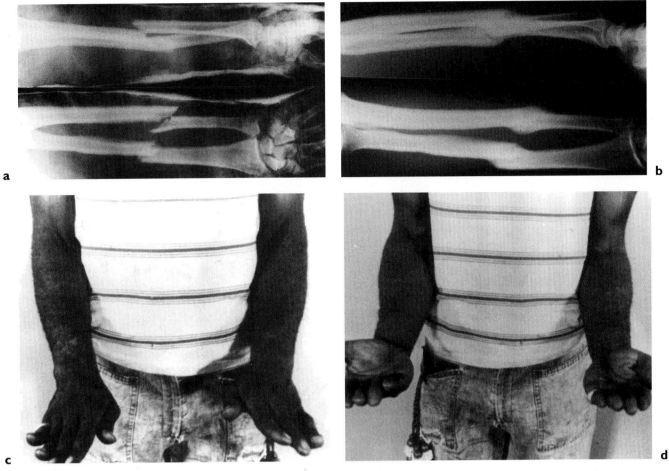

FIGURE 4.22.   Closed oblique fractures of both bones of the forearm are shown. Notice the mild shortening of the extremity and the overriding of the fragments (**A**). The fracture was treated with a functional brace that permitted motion of the elbow and flexion and extension of the wrist. The fractures healed without additional shortening and acceptable alignment (**B**). Fractures that are oblique in nature and with overriding fragments constitute the ideal fractures for functional bracing. Additional shortening does not take place, and the ultimate loss of pronosupination is minimal and comparable with that obtained after successful surgical plating. The patient demonstrates the final range of motion of his forearm, which was limited only in the last few degrees of pronation (**C** and **D**).

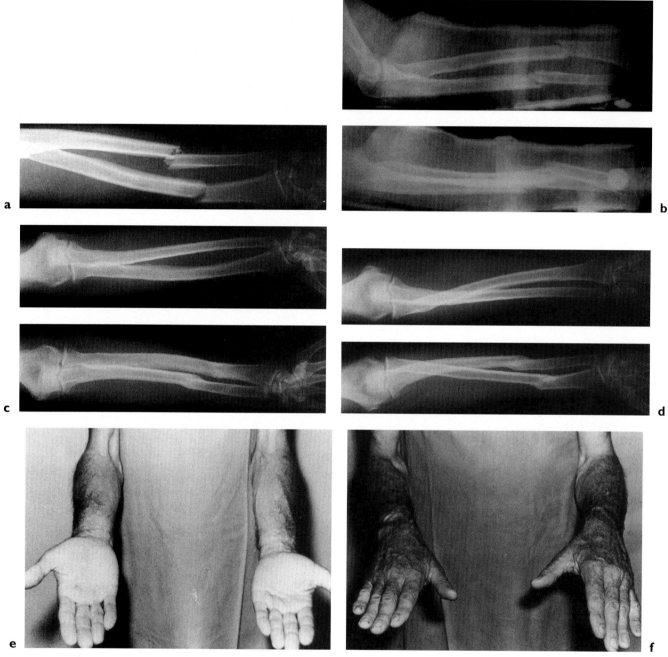

FIGURE 4.23. Closed oblique fractures of both bones of the forearm are shown (**A**). Acceptable alignment of the fragments was obtained by simply hanging the arm with Chinese fingertraps for approximately 10 minutes (**B**). The fractures healed with very satisfactory range of motion of the forearm. The radiographs depict the extreme degrees of pronosupination of both forearms (**C and D**). The patient demonstrates the permanent mild limitation of pronation. The patient compensates very inconspicuously for this limitation by shoulder flexion and internal rotation (**E and F**).

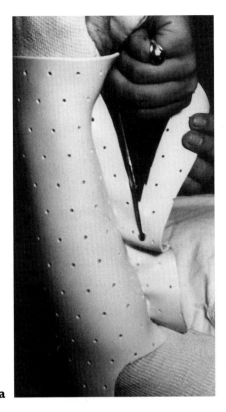

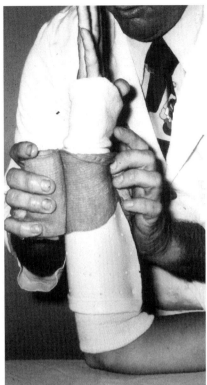

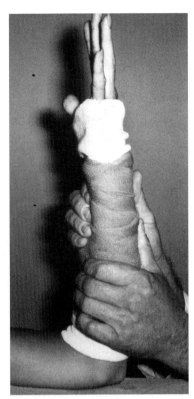

a

b, c

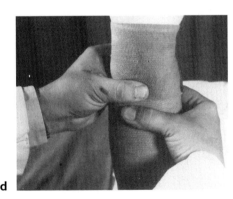

d

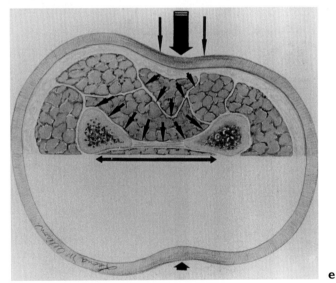

e

FIGURE 4.24. Steps to be taken during the fabrication of a functional Orthoplast brace: A sheet of Orthoplast is wrapped over the extremity, extending from 2 in above the elbow to just below the wrist (**A**). The soft and pliable sheet is then firmly wrapped with an elastic bandage saturated in cold water (**B**). As the plastic material begins to set, the dorsal and volar aspect of the forearm is firmly compressed, attempting to separate the two bones as much as possible (**C and D**). During the entire procedure, the forearm is held in a relaxed attitude of supination. The drawing depicts the effect of compression of the soft tissues and the resulting separation between the two bones (**E**).

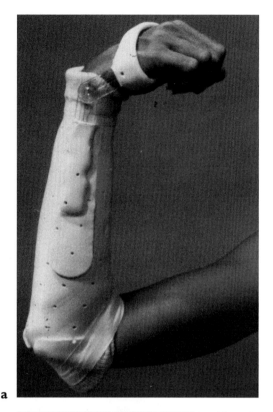

a

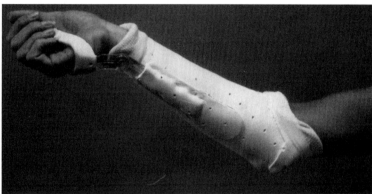

b

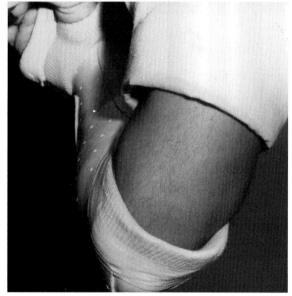

c

FIGURE 4.25. The completed Orthoplast brace demonstrates the mild limitation of elbow flexion (**A**), the lack of extension in the last 30 degrees (**B**), and the free flexion and extension of the wrist. The proximal posterior extension of the brace over the olecranon and the firm compression over the supracondylar region prevent pronation and supination of the forearm (**C and D**). *Continued.*

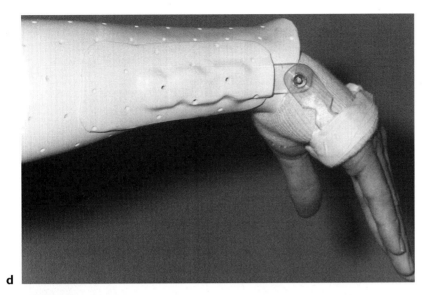

d

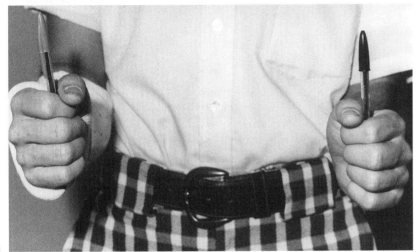

e

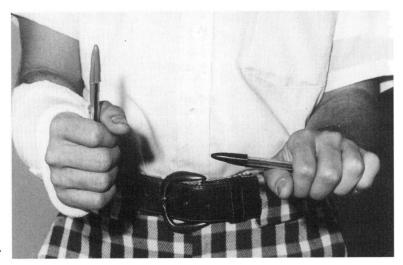

f

FIGURE 4.25. *Continued*   The patient demonstrates how the brace permits only a few degrees of pronation and supination of the forearm (**E and F**).

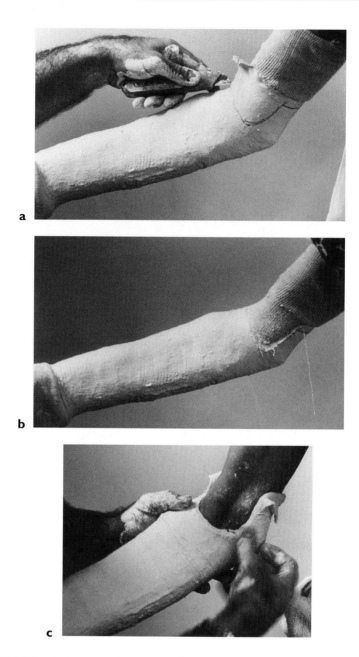

FIGURE 4.26. In the event the treating physician does not have the Orthoplast material available, plaster of Paris can be used. The forearm, as in the case of bracing using plastic materials, is held in a relaxed attitude of supination. Plaster is wrapped over the elbow, and the supracondylar region is firmly compressed. The volar and dorsal surfaces of the forearm are firmly flattened. The anterior wall of the cast over the elbow is trimmed to permit eventual flexion of the elbow. The stockinet is folded over the sharp edges of the plaster (**A–C**).

The combined loss of pronosupination in the patient with the fractures located in the proximal third of the forearm was 11 degrees. The 28 patients with fractures in the middle third of the forearm lost an average of 13 degrees of pronosupination. The 10 patients with fractures in the distal third lost an average of 8 degrees of pronosupination.

BASIC GUIDELINES FOR PHYSICIANS

Guidelines for physicians using functional braces in the categories discussed in this chapter may be found in the many publications listed in References.

REFERENCES

1. Bowker P, Pratt DJ, McLaughlan J, et al. Early weight-bearing treatment of femoral shaft fractures using a cast-brace: a preliminary biomechanical study. *J Bioeng* 1978;2:463.
2. Bunger C, Solund K, Rasmussen P. Early results after Colles' fractures: functional bracing in supination versus dorsal plaster immobilization. *Arch Orthop Trauma Surg* 1984; 103:25.
3. Connolly JF, Dehne E, LaFollette B. Closed reduction and early cast brace ambulation in the treatment of femoral fractures. *J Bone Joint Surg (Am)* 1973;55:1581.
4. Connolly JF, Dehne E, LaFollette B. Closed revision and early cast brace ambulation in the treatment of femoral fractures. *J Bone Joint Surg (Am)* 1978;60:112.
5. DeLee JC, Clanton TO, Rockwood CA. Closed treatment of subtrochanteric fractures of the femur in a modified cast-brace. *J Bone Joint Surg (Am)* 1979;63:135.
6. Frykman G. Fractures of the distal radius including sequelae: shoulder-hand-finger syndrome, disturbance of the distal radioulnar joint and impairment of nerve function. A clinical and experimental study. *Acta Orthop Scand [Suppl]* 1967;108:1–155.
7. Gross RH, Davidson R, Sullivan JA, et al. Cast brace management of the femoral shaft fracture in children and young adults. *J Pediatr Orthop* 1983;3:572.
8. Hackethorm JC, Burkhalter WE, Donley JM, et al. Review of 156 open femoral fractures. Treatment with traction and cast bracing. *J Bone Joint Surg (Am)* 1975;57:1029.
9. Hardy AE. Pressure recording in patients with femoral fractures in cast-braces and suggestions for treatment. *J Bone Joint Surg (Am)* 1982;61:365.
10. Hardy AE. The treatment of femoral fractures by cast-brace application and early ambulation—a prospective review of one hundred and six patients. *J Bone Joint Surg (Am)* 1983;65:56.
11. Iwegbu CG. Preliminary results of treatment of fractures of the femur by cast-bracing using the Zaria metal hinge. *Injury* 1984;15:250.
12. Kristensen KD, Kiaer T, Blicher J. No arthrosis of the ankle 20 years after malaligned tibial-shaft fracture. *Acta Orthop Scand* 1989;60:208.
13. Kumar R. Treatment of fracture of the femur in children by a "cast brace." *Int Surg* 1982;67(suppl 4):551–552.
14. Linson MA, Lewinnek F, White AA. Ischemic complications of femoral cast-bracing: report of two cases. *Clin Orthop* 1982;162:189.
15. Llinas A, McKellop H, Marshall J, et al. Healing and remodeling of articular incongruities in a rabbit fracture model. *J Bone Joint Surg (Am)* 1993;75:1508–1523.
16. Lovasz G, Llinas A, Benya P, et al. Effects of valgus tibial angulation on cartilage degeneration in the rabbit knee. *J Orthop Res* 1995;13:846–853.
17. Lovasz G, Park SH, Ebramzadeh E, et al. Characteristics of degeneration in an unstable knee with a coronal surface step-off. *J Bone Joint Surg (Br)* 2001;82:428–436.
18. McCollough NC, Vinsant JE, Sarmiento A. Functional fracture-bracing of long-bone fractures of the lower extremity in children. *J Bone Joint Surg (Am)* 1978;60:314.
19. Meggitt BF, Vaughan-Lane T. Hip hinge thigh brace for early mobilization of proximal femoral shaft fractures. *Prosthet Orthot Int* 1980;4:150.
20. Mooney V, Nickel VL, Harvey JP, et al. Cast-brace treatment for fractures of the distal part of the femur. *J Bone Joint Surg (Am)* 1970;52:1563.
21. Moore TM, Lester DK, Sarmiento A. The stabilizing effect of soft-tissue constraints in the artificial Galeazzi fractures. *Clin Orthop* 1985;194:189.
22. Rankin EA, Metz CW. Management of delayed union in early weight-bearing treatment of the fractured tibia. *J Trauma* 1970;10:751.
23. Sarmiento A. Application of prosthetic principles to fracture care. *Spectator Lett* 1963.
24. Sarmiento A. The brachioradialis as a deforming force in Colles' fractures. *Clin Orthop* 1965;38:86.
25. Sarmiento A. Functional bracing of tibial and femoral shaft fractures. *Clin Orthop* 1972; 82:2.
26. Sarmiento A, Burkhalter W, Latta LL. Functional bracing in the management of aseptic delayed union and nonunion of the tibial diaphysis. (in press).
27. Sarmiento A, Cooper JS, Sinclair WF. Forearm fractures. Early functional bracing—a preliminary report. *J Bone Joint Surg (Am)* 1975;57:297.
28. Sarmiento A, Ebramzadeh E, Brys D, et al. Angular deformities and forearm fractures. *J Orthop Res* 1992;10:121–133.
29. Sarmiento A, Latta LL. *The closed functional treatment of fractures.* Heidelberg: Springer-Verlag, 1981.

30. Sarmiento A. Closed treatment of distal radius fractures. *Techniques in Orthopaedics* 2000;15:294–304.
31. Sarmiento A, Pratt GW, Berry NC, et al. Colles' fractures—functional bracing in supination. *J Bone Joint Surg (Am)* 1975;57:311.
32. Sarmiento A, Zagorski JB, Sinclair WF. Functional bracing of Colles' fractures: a prospective study of immobilization in supination vs. pronation. *Clin Orthop* 1980;146:175.
33. Smail GB. Long term follow-up of Colles' fractures. *J Bone Joint Surg (Br)* 1965;47:80–85.
34. Stewart HD, Innes AR, Burke FD. Functional cast-bracing for Colles' fractures: a comparison between cast-bracing and conventional plaster casts. *J Bone Joint Surg (Br)* 1984;66:749.
35. Tarr R, Garfinkle A, Sarmiento A. The effects of angular deformity of both bones of the forearm: an in-vivo study. *J Bone Joint Surg (Am)* 1984;66:65–70.
36. Thomas TL, Meggitt BF. A comparative study of methods for treating fractures of the distal half of the femur. *J Bone Joint Surg (Br)* 1981;63:3.
37. Wardlaw D, McLaughlan J, Pratt DJ, et al. A biomechanical study of cast-brace treatment of femoral shaft fractures. *J Bone Joint Surg (Br)* 1981;63:7.
38. Zagorski JB, Zych GA, Latta LL, et al. Management of Colles' fractures with pre-fabricated braces. *Orthop Trans* 1986;10:471.
39. Zagorski JB, Zych GA, Latta LL, et al. Modern concepts in functional fracture bracing—upper limb. In: *AAOS instructional course lectures, 36.* Chicago: American Academy of Orthopaedic Surgeons, 1987.

Subject Index

Page numbers followed by *f* indicate figures.

A

Angular deformities
    clinical significance, 3, 7–8*f*
    femoral shaft fracture outcomes, 157
    forearm fracture outcomes, 163–164
    humeral shaft fracture outcomes, 12,
        14–16*ff*, 19*f*, 21*f*, 30*f*, 33, 38*f*,
        40*f*, 45*f*, 46–48*ff*, 50–51*f*, 52*f*,
        54, 56–58*ff*, 60
    humeral tolerance, 12, 54, 61
    tibial shaft fracture outcomes, 82–83,
        86–91*ff*, 92, 97*f*, 98*f*, 105*f*, 108,
        110*f*, 111*f*, 135, 138, 139
    tibial tolerance, 83, 102
    ulnar shaft fracture outcomes, 66,
        72*f*, 74*f*
Arthritis. *See* Joint disease, postfracture

B

Brace application and maintenance
    Colles' fracture treatment, 151, 154*f*
    femoral shaft treatment, 157
    forearm fracture treatment, 164,
        167–170*ff*
    humeral shaft fracture treatment, 12,
        33–34, 35, 41–42*f*, 43*f*, 61, 62
    soft plaster, 34
    tibial shaft fracture treatment, 82,
        102, 103–108, 106*f*, 118–119,
        125–133*ff*, 134–135,
        136–137*ff*, 138, 139
        below-the-knee functional cast,
            109–118, 116*f*
    ulnar shaft fracture treatment, 67, 68,
        69, 70–71*f*, 75, 77, 78

C

Cast
    forearm fracture treatment, 164
    humeral shaft stabilization, 13,
        24–25*f*, 34
    soft plaster, 34
    tibial shaft
        below-the-knee, 109–118,
            120–124*ff*
        stabilization, 90*f*, 92–93, 102, 103,
            109
    ulnar shaft fracture treatment, 66, 67
Colles' fracture
    articular incongruity in, 156
    electrical stimulation, 153*f*

functional bracing of, 150–151,
    152–155*ff*, 155–156, 158–159*ff*
    manipulative reduction, 152*f*, 154*f*
    with radioulnar joint dislocation,
        153*f*, 158*f*
    treatment goals, 151
    treatment selection, 3, 144, 150
Cost of care, 2–3, 9
    causes of increases in, 144–145
    femoral shaft bracing, 157
    humeral shaft fracture treatment, 60
    tibial shaft fracture treatment, 135
    ulnar fracture fixation, 76

D

Diaphyseal fractures
    indications for functional bracing, 8–9
    nonunion/delayed union, 55
    See also Humeral shaft fracture;
        Tibial shaft fracture; Ulnar shaft
        fracture

E

Exercise regimen
    humeral shaft fracture treatment, 13,
        33, 34–35, 42*f*, 44*f*, 61, 62
    tibia shaft fracture treatment,
        101–102, 109
    ulnar shaft fracture treatment, 75

F

Femoral shaft fracture, functional
        bracing of, 156–157, 159–162*ff*,
        162
Fibula fracture
    concurrent tibia fracture, 85*f*, 86*f*, 92,
        94*f*, 97*f*, 98*f*, 110*f*, 111*f*, 135
    postfracture shortening, 5–6*f*
Forearm
    fractures of both bones, 163–164,
        165–170*ff*, 170
    plate fixation, 3
Functional fracture bracing
    of Colles' fracture, 150–151,
        152–155*ff*, 155–156
    of femoral fractures, 156–157,
        159–162*ff*, 162
    of fractures of both forearm bones,
        163–164, 165–170*ff*
    historical development, 2, 144
    indications, 8–9

rationale, 2, 144
    shortening outcomes, 4*f*, 5–6*f*
    for tibial nonunion/delayed union,
        145, 146–149*ff*, 150
    See also Humeral shaft fracture;
        Tibial shaft fracture; Ulnar shaft
        fracture

H

Humeral shaft fracture, functional
        bracing of
    acute management, 12–13
    alignment outcomes, 17–18*f*, 19*f*, 20*f*,
        22*f*, 25–28*ff*, 36–37*f*, 38*f*, 40*f*,
        48*f*, 54–55
    angular deformities after, 3, 7–8*f*, 12,
        14–16*f*, 19–21*ff*, 30*f*, 33, 38*f*,
        40*f*, 45–48*ff*, 50–51*f*, 52*f*,
        56–58*ff*, 60, 61
    with axial distraction, 13, 31–32*f*, 55
    brace application and maintenance,
        12, 33–34, 35, 41–42*f*, 43*f*, 55,
        61, 62
    with brachial plexus injury, 13
    carrying angle outcomes, 37*f*, 45*f*,
        51*f*, 54, 56*f*
    causes of malalignment, 54–55
    clinical guidelines, 61
    closed fracture, 12–13, 33
    comminuted fracture, 13, 14*f*,
        19–22*ff*, 27–30*ff*, 36–37*f*, 40*f*,
        45*f*, 49*f*, 50*f*, 52*f*, 54–55
    compartment syndromes, 13
    contraindications, 12, 61
    cost of care, 60
    distal extraarticular, 36*f*
    exercise regimen, 13, 33, 34–35, 42*f*,
        44*f*, 61, 62
    indications, 12, 61
    joint contracture complications, 33
    manipulation of limb during, 33, 54
    medial butterfly fragment, 36*f*
    nerve palsy complications, 33,
        36–37*f*, 54
    nonunion/delayed union, 55, 60
    oblique fracture of distal third,
        17–18*f*, 48*f*
    oblique fracture of middle third,
        15–16*f*
    open fracture, 13
    outcomes, 35, 60

Humeral shaft fracture, functional
    bracing of (contd.)
  patient self-care, 12, 34–35, 62
  plate fixation, 13, 32f
  posttrauma stabilization, 13, 23–24f,
      33
  range of motion outcomes, 55–60, 59f
  rationale, 12
  refractures, 49f, 50f, 55, 60
  rotary deformity, 43f
  segmental fractures, 13, 21f, 22f
  shoulder subluxation in, 33, 36f, 60
  skin problems during, 55
  transverse middle, 38f, 50f, 51f

I

Incongruous joints, 3–8
Internal fixation
  cost of care, 2–3
  femoral shaft fractures, 156, 157
  of forearm fractures, 163
  indications, 150
  rationale, 3

J

Joint disease, postfracture
  angular deformities, 3
  Colles' fracture and, 151
  incongruity effects, 3–8, 156
  tibial shaft fracture outcomes, 103

M

Monteggia fracture, 66

N

Nerve palsies
  as humeral shaft fracture
      complication, 33, 36–37f, 54
  tibial shaft fracture outcomes,
      103–108

O

Ostectomy
  to stimulate osteogenesis, 145
  in tibial functional bracing for
      nonunion, 145, 146f, 148–149ff
Osteogenesis, 145
Outcomes
  angular deformities, 3, 7–8f
  clinical conceptualization, 3, 150, 151
  Colles' fracture treatment, 151,
      155–156
  femoral shaft fractures, 157–162,
      159f, 160f, 161f
  fracture of both forearm bones, 164,
      165f, 166f, 170
  humeral shaft fractures, 13, 14–23ff,
      26–32ff, 35, 36–41ff, 45–53ff,
      54–60
  joint incongruity, 3–8
  postfracture shortening, 2, 3, 4f, 5–6f
  of surgical interventions, 2–9, 144

tibial functional bracing for
    nonunion, 150
tibial shaft fracture, 84–91ff,
    94–101ff, 102–103, 104–107ff,
    110–115ff
ulnar shaft fracture, 68, 71–74ff,
    75–76, 77

P

Plate fixation
  for Colles' fracture, 150
  forearm, 3
  of forearm fractures, 163
  humeral shaft fracture, 13, 32f
  outcomes, 3
  for ulnar shaft fracture, 66

R

Rigid fracture fixation
  clinical goals, 3
  problems of, 2–3
  rationale, 2, 3
Rotary deformities
  clinical significance, 3
  forearm fracture outcomes, 163
  humeral shaft fracture outcomes, 55,
      60
  mechanism, 43f
  tibial shaft fracture outcomes, 103,
      107f, 119–134
  ulnar shaft fracture outcomes, 66

S

Shortening of fractured bone
  clinical conceptualization, 2, 3, 4f,
      150
  Colles' fracture, 156
  forearm fracture, 165f
  tibial fracture, 82, 83, 84f, 92, 95f,
      102, 108, 135, 138, 139
  ulnar fracture, 76
Skin problems, 55, 69
Sling, for humeral shaft stabilization, 13,
    24–25f, 35
Splint
  humeral shaft stabilization, 13, 24f
  ulnar shaft fracture treatment, 67
Surgical interventions, 2–9, 144, 150,
    151
Synostosis, as ulnar shaft fracture
    complication, 68–69, 76

T

Tibial shaft fracture, functional bracing
    of
  acute management, 92–93
  angular deformities in, 82–83,
      84–91ff, 92, 95–98ff, 102, 105f,
      108, 110f, 111f, 135, 138, 139
  axial instability, 82, 83, 135
  brace application and maintenance,
      102, 103–108, 106f, 138

below-the-knee functional cast,
    109, 116f, 117–118, 120–124ff
custom-made brace, 118–119,
    125–132ff
function, 82, 118
patient instructions, 139
prefabricated brace, 119, 133f,
    134–135, 136–137ff
clinical guidelines, 138
closed fractures, 92–93
comminuted fracture, 87f, 91f, 94f,
    95f, 98f, 104–107ff, 110f, 113f,
    115f
compartment syndrome risk, 101
concurrent fibular fracture, 85f, 86f,
    92, 94f, 97f, 98f, 110f, 111f,
    135
contraindications, 83, 92, 97f, 135,
    138
cost of care, 135
exercise regimen, 101–102, 109
expected outcomes, 102–103, 135
gender differences, 83
indications, 83, 92, 135, 138
with intraarticular incongruity, 108,
    113–115ff
manipulation of limb, 93, 101
nail fixation and, 83–92, 108, 112f
nerve palsy related to, 103–108
nonunion/delayed union, 102, 108,
    135, 145, 146–149ff, 150
oblique fractures, 97f
open fractures, 93, 103, 104–106ff
patient instructions, 101–102,
    134–135, 139
postfracture shortening, 4f, 5–6f, 82,
    83, 84f, 92, 95f, 102, 108, 135,
    138, 139
range of motion outcomes, 103, 115f
rationale, 82–83
recurvatum risk, 83, 90f, 91f,
    109–117
rotary deformities, 103, 107f,
    119–134
segmental fractures, 93, 96f, 99f,
    100f, 101f, 102, 112f
stabilization cast, 90f, 92–93, 102,
    103, 109

U

Ulnar shaft fracture, functional bracing
    of
  acute management, 67
  angular deformity in, 66, 72f, 74f
  brace application and maintenance,
      67, 68, 69, 70–71f, 75, 77, 78
  callus formation, 68, 69, 71f, 74f
  casts, 66, 67
  clinical guidelines, 77
  closed fractures, 67
  comminuted fracture, 73f

contraindications, 66, 77
cost of care, 76
exercise regimen, 75
forearm prosupination, 67, 72f, 73f, 75, 77
indications, 66, 77
malalignment, 69

Monteggia type, 66
muscular weakness in, 69
nonunion/delayed union, 69
open fractures, 66, 67
outcomes, 68, 75–76, 77
patient self-care, 68, 78
versus plate fixation, 66

posttrauma stabilization, 67
range of motion outcomes, 68, 69–75, 77, 78
rationale, 66
refracture, 69
skin problems in, 69
synostosis risk, 68–69, 76